In God's Hand

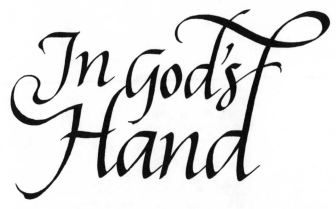

In God's Hand

One Woman's Experience
with Breast Cancer

Becky Lynn Wecksler and Michael Wecksler

HERALD PRESS
Scottdale, Pennsylvania
Kitchener, Ontario

Library of Congress Cataloging-in-Publication Data

Wecksler, Becky Lynn, 1951-
    In God's hand.

    1. Wecksler, Becky Lynn, 1951-   —Health.
2. Breast—Cancer—Patients—California—Biography.
3. Christian life—1960-   I. Wecksler, Michael,
1953-   II. Title.
RC280.B8W389   1989   362.1'9699449'00924 [B]   88-35807
ISBN 0-8361-3492-3 (alk. paper)

The paper used in this publication meets the minimum requirements of
American National Standard for Information Sciences—Permanence of Paper for
Printed Library Materials, ANSI Z39.48-1984.

Except as otherwise indicated, Scripture quotations are from the *Holy Bible: New
International Version.* Copyright © 1973, 1978, 1984 by the International Bible
Society. Used by permission of Zondervan Bible Publishers.

95   94   93   92   91   90   89   10   9   8   7   6   5   4   3   2   1

To David, Stephen, Aaron and Aimee. I am so glad that God chose me to be your mother and let me live so that I might watch you grow. Along with Wayne, my beloved husband. You have always been and will always be my love.

Contents

Foreword by Stephnee K. Grainger .9
Author's Preface 11
Acknowledgments 13

1. Is It Cancer? 17
2. Suspicion Confirmed 27
3. A Black Cloud 36
4. Prayers of Faith 42
5. A Daze of Consultations 47
6. Gathering Strength 54
7. Trauma and Trust 62
8. The Chemotherapy Ordeal 71
9. Pac Men, Fire, and Water 86
10. On to Recovery 96

The Authors 101

Foreword

I was still in the dark fog of the anesthesia after my breast biopsy. Through the hum of the machinery and the bustle of nursing activity my surgeon's voice suddenly boomed loudly in my ear. "You have cancer. The tumor was huge. Massive." Two weeks later I was back in the hospital for a modified radical mastectomy. I was 33 years old.

As a registered nurse I specialized in counseling cancer patients and their families. As a minister's daughter, I had a strong faith in the power of God. I was supported by my husband, children, relatives and friends. I believed that I was uniquely prepared to successfully cope with the changes that would take place in my life. Imagine my surprise when I discovered that cancer was not the manageable affair I thought it would be!

Perhaps, like me, you believe you have the personal strength to cope with cancer alone. As I read *In God's Hand* I was reminded how thoroughly I had fooled myself following my mastectomy. The human mind cannot help but worry over the recurrence of cancer, mourn the disfigurement that results, envy those women who still have two normal breasts, and feel that life will never be happy again. Like Becky, I wondered why this horrible disease had to happen to me. I found little pleasure in the wonder of life about me and felt completely justified in all my self-pity.

In God's Hand affirms what we, as Christians, should already know—that we cannot possibly handle cancer, or any major life crisis, all by ourselves. Sooner or later we must all relinquish the desire to guide our lives by our own thoughts alone. *In God's Hand* reminds us that God is always waiting patiently to take the burden of fear and doubt from our shoulders. It is not a sign of weakness to say, "God, I can't handle this all by myself. Please help me." Rather, it is a sign of strength, a belief in the promise of faith as taught us by Jesus, that the healing power of God's love will work miracles in our lives if we only allow his presence into our hearts.

The message of faith contained within these pages goes far beyond medical cure of disease. If we turn from God because we have not been completely cured of illness, we cheat ourselves, not realizing God's true promise. Coping with serious illness is only one way in which we gain the opportunity to come closer to God's love. It is not the triumph of the body over disease that proves God works his miracles in our lives, but the triumph of the spirit over doubt and despair. *In God's Hand* testifies that by allowing God to carry us through adversity we will be rewarded with the true gift we seek as Christians—the healing of the eternal soul.

Stephnee K. Grainger, RN, BSN
Ventura, California
September 1988

Author's Preface

In God's Hand comes from the true experiences of my life after being diagnosed as having breast cancer. During the course of my illness, I constantly felt the need to know how others like myself handled the daily demands of life as mother, wife, and working woman. I was hungry for an autobiography of someone who was not famous or wealthy, someone that I could relate to. I needed to know if my fears and feelings were the same as those experienced by other women with this disease.

This book was prepared to help others with cancer—others who share those same fears and feelings. It was written to help them see, through my life, that there is hope, that there are things they can personally do to help get them through the tough times, and that their own response may actually help the healing process.

Our nature is to want to control our own destiny. Most of us live as if we believe that we really do. We place our confidence in ourselves and in what we can accomplish on our own effort. We believe we need no hands but our own. For many, it takes the fear that our lives are slipping from our hands for us to begin to question this presumption and search for a higher meaning. And when we do, we find that there is one hand that is always stretched out to take ours. God's hand.

> To touch one life,
> To ease her way,
> To share God's light,
> For this I pray.

> *Becky Lynn Wecksler*
> *Saugus, California*
> *September 1988*

Acknowledgments

This book would still be just another silent experience if it had not been for the encouragement of my mother-in-law, Gladys Wecksler, who insisted that I keep a diary of my ordeal, and my brother-in-law, Michael Wecksler, who asked if he could put my story into print. These special people, and many others, I would like to thank.

The first is my husband, Wayne, for his love, patience, and steadfast support. I could not have made it without his positive attitude and strength to hold me together when I no longer had the courage to continue. My mother, Pat McIntyre, and Gladys Wecksler, who faithfully came to help when I was not capable of caring for my family. They were angels of mercy, sensing my needs and keeping our house a home when life was in disarray.

I would like to thank my sisters, Cheryl Spiro and Susan Kane, and my sister-in-law Charlotte Wecksler, who kept a vigil by my bedside during my surgeries and were always there for me with a listening ear and an open heart.

Throughout my illness, many good friends sent their love, prayers and support. Among those were Buzz and

Tina Brown, Cathy and Gary Leason, Jim and Melanie Thomas, Nate and Evelyn Thomas, Glenn and Tilda Goodwin, Geri and Steve Hacket, Linda and John Hayward, Stephnee Grainger, Betty Gartner, Florence Galloway, Evelyn Okert, Larry and Cathy Brooks, Larry and Debbie Morse, and David and Laurie Mefford.

I want to give an acknowledgment to Terri Lauricella, who has gone home to be with the Lord, and Jeannie Cooper; through their own tremendous faith and struggles with cancer, they gave me courage and inspiration.

Thanks are due to the many friends from Faith Community Church for all their love, prayers, and support. I especially want to thank Kathleen McCulloch, Val Hitchcock, Sherry McDiffett, Kim Bowers, Jim and Emily Frost, Alan and Debbie Burdette, Janice Gentry, and Jeanette Clark. God showed me what being a servant was through their actions.

I also want to give a heartfelt thanks to my hairdresser, Susie Panda. At one of my lowest points, she created a hairstyle for me that bolstered my confidence and allowed me to go out in public without a wig.

My coworkers at Henry Mayo Newhall Memorial Hospital were highly supportive in easing me back into my old job. They included Kathy Parkin, Pam Borrelli, Gayle Oliphant, Rosanne Voorhees, Anne Sweatnam, Becky Lebben, Carol Leahy, Vivian Whitman, and Nancy Freund.

Finally, I would like to express my deepest appreciation to the staff at the Breast Center, Dr. James Waisman, Dr. Melvin Silverstein, Dr. Parvis Gamagami, Dr. Neal Handel, Ellen Waisman, B.S., and Sherry LeDuc, R.N., for their expertise in my care.

Becky Lynn Wecksler

In God's Hand

1

Is It Cancer?

The doctor and I were standing in front of a lighted viewing screen looking at the X-rays of my breasts when the words that would shake my world to its foundation boomed inside my head.

"I think it's cancer, Mrs. Wecksler."

"What?" I asked, dumbfounded.

"I think you have a case of early cancer," he said, pointing with a pencil at a small "wheel" of calcification at the bottom base of my left breast. "But you're lucky. We've caught it at an early stage. We'll probably remove the mass and then put you on radiation therapy for a while, but I think you'll be fine."

A thick fog settled on my mind and all the primitive fears of an unseen foe began to well up within me. "How much radiation?" I managed to ask.

"I'm not sure, but probably only a few weeks. We'll see."

It occurred to me that Dr. Gamagami was either a skilled, confident diagnostician, or a fool for scaring me without a reason. I quickly realized he was not a fool.

I had discovered the lumps on my breast a few weeks before, while lying in bed next to my husband, Wayne. My left breast was tender, and as I gently massaged it I felt two lumps: one on the top and one on the side next to the chest wall. Wayne assured me that I had always had those lumps and that they were nothing to worry about, but I was unconvinced. I had felt them before, of course, but I had always assumed—along with the doctors I had visited— that the lumps were merely swollen milk glands that would shrink as soon as I quit breast-feeding. Though I had breast-fed all four of my young children, I had not done so in over two years. Something was definitely wrong.

My discovery was still on my mind the next morning as I drove to work. During the fifteen-minute drive from my home in Saugus to the Henry Mayo Medical Center in Valencia, where I worked as a nurse, my mind reeled with self-concern. Why didn't I think about the lumps before? Why didn't the doctors discover them in my numerous exams? I thought back to a conversation I had overheard in the hospital cafeteria a few weeks before.

A woman at the table next to me was telling her companions about a friend of hers who had died of breast cancer.

"I tell you," she had said in a high-pitched voice, "her husband is a doctor, and he should have known she had cancer. I think he knew and didn't tell her because he wanted her family's money."

I remembered thinking at the time that the woman was absurd and suspicious. I had felt comfort in the fact that my husband certainly loved me too much to do something like that. Of course, I assumed then that a husband would be able to tell if his wife began to develop lumps in her breast. I later learned that they rarely do.

When I got to work I told some nurses on my floor about the lumps. Since we had recently moved to Saugus from the Bay Area, I didn't know any gynecologists. I asked them to make a recommendation. I made an appointment with a doctor in Valencia and waited anxiously for a few days before I could get in.

The doctor told me the lumps were probably just cysts and that I didn't have breast cancer. He said I should have a mammogram—an X-ray of the breast—to begin a baseline from which one could measure any changes in the tissue. He recommended the mammogram be done at The Breast Center in Van Nuys and scheduled an appointment for me.

The next twelve days were fine. My world revolved once again around my family, my life, and my work. All the fear was washed from my mind and an almost physical burden was lifted from me. I was once again my usual happy-go-lucky self.

That feeling stayed with me as I drove to The Breast Center. I made my way through the heavy Los Angeles traffic with little concern. When I entered the facility, which occupied the entire sixth floor of a medical building, I felt as if everything was going to be all right.

I was relaxed and unconcerned as I stared at the smoggy view of Van Nuys through a picture window in the waiting room. I told myself I'd just be given some routine checks and be on my way home. I wondered if the other women in the waiting room had breast cancer and felt separated from them because I was only there for tests. It was a feeling that would soon disappear.

A female technician called my name and led me to an

examining room. She instructed me to strip to the waist and place my breasts, one at a time, between the two plates of the mammography machine. We joked easily as she took a number of X-rays from different angles, but after she returned from viewing them in a separate room, the mood suddenly changed.

Dr. Gamagami, with a quizzical look on his face, followed the technician into the room. He put both hands on my back and gently pushed, forcing my chest wall up against the plates of the machine. The technician then took another X-ray.

By the time they had finished, my tepidity had turned to anxiety. Why were they so quiet? What were they whispering about? Why were they talking as if I were just an object?

The technician told me I needed another test. She told me to dress and then led me down the hall to a closet-like room for a thermogram. I was told to strip to the waist again, put my hands on my head, and face what looked like a video camera. The room was chilled in order to make the thermogram more effective, and I sat in the cold wondering what was going on. After the doctor and technician left I chuckled at the thought that there might be a peephole somewhere in the wall, with someone looking at me while I sat naked from the waist up, facing a video camera with my hands on my head like a German soldier surrendering to the Allied forces. I couldn't imagine what all the concern was. After all, didn't I just have some cysts? Maybe they were bigger than the doctors thought.

After the thermogram, the technician led me to a viewing screen where Dr. Gamagami waited to show me my film.

"Mrs. Wecksler, your lumps are nothing," he said, looking at the film with a magnifying glass.

I was relieved to hear that my gynecologist was right after all. But what about all the concern the doctor and technician had shown? I didn't have to wait long to find out.

"But right here," he said, showing me on the X-ray a small spot on the bottom of my breast, "we have a little area of calcification. It's very small and I almost missed it. That's why we had a thermogram, which shows warm areas of the breast. If an area is warm, then there's an increase in vascularity, an increase in activity. It's like a red flag, something we should keep an eye on." He stood back from the screen for a moment. "But even if I had not found the calcification I would have had you come back in six months." He explained that the entire breast was warm but that the lumps were not unusually warm. He told me emphatically that the wheel of calcification appeared cancerous.

He handed me the magnifying glass and I stared at the round cluster of cancer cells. He said I should select a surgeon and that nothing further could be determined until the surgeon made a diagnosis, but I wasn't listening. All I could think about was how my life had suddenly become endangered. I marveled at the fact that something so small could radically alter my life and perhaps end it. Fear began to press down on me like a stone.

"I think everything will be all right, Becky. After all, it's just a small area, and with the lumpectomy and radiation therapy, there's every reason to believe that all the cancerous tissue will be removed or destroyed," the doctor said reassuringly as they led me out of the viewing room.

We walked silently back to the lobby where I had sat so smugly just an hour earlier. In a daze, I picked up one of the surgeons' cards from the reception desk and walked out the door. Ignoring the elevators, I walked down the six flights of stairs and out into the hot September sun.

I knew I was in no shape to make the 45-minute drive to my home in Saugus, so I called my mother, hoping she would help me steady myself. "Honey, they won't know anything until they do a biopsy, so don't you worry," she assured me. "Everything's going to be just fine, Beck. Do you want me to come and get you?"

I smiled at the thought of waiting an hour-and-a-half while my mother drove to Van Nuys from Riverside in heavy traffic to drive me home.

"No, Mom. I'll be all right," I lied to her. "Don't worry. I just had to tell someone about all this."

I hung up the phone, walked to my car, and drove home in tears. I was scheduled to work that night, but I called and told them what had happened. I didn't think I would be very effective in such a state of mind. Besides, I wanted to be there when Wayne got home so I could tell him what we were about to face.

I didn't tell the children what was wrong with me, though I suspect they knew something was up. I did the laundry, cleaned the house, fed the kids and put them to bed, and then waited quietly for Wayne to get home that evening. In addition to working as a biochemist, he was taking night classes at UCLA for his master's degree in business administration. Two times a week he came in after nine o'clock. The minute he came through the door, I burst into tears.

"Oh, honey," I sobbed, hugging him before he had a

chance to put down his briefcase. "They discovered a couple of lumps and a cluster of calcification. The lumps are benign, but they think the cluster is cancerous."

He exhaled loudly and hugged me tightly. Then he held me at arm's length. The color had drained from his face and he was tight-lipped, but he spoke calmly and without a great deal of emotion.

He was surprised, of course, and asked me how they knew I had a problem. I told him about the procedure and what would come next. He smiled at me thinly and held me again.

"Well, let's just wait and see what's going to happen. We're not sure of anything right now, and there's no sense getting all worked up before we know there's a problem."

I began to give in to his stoic mood. "He did say it was in its early stages and could be treated with just a lumpectomy and radiation," I said. "It might be nothing."

"Well, that's right. It may not be serious at all. If it is, we'll deal with it as the time comes. Right now we don't know anything for sure." He held me tightly again and I felt his strength rush through my body. I was very grateful for having him. If Wayne had reacted in any other way, I don't know what I would have done. He had always been a source of strength for me, and always would be. He kissed me and then went into the kitchen and got us each a drink. We sat on the living-room couch as we tried to talk of other things. After a while we went up to bed, where we both lay quietly and thought about the one thing neither of us wanted to think about.

From that point on I began to view the world with a new set of eyes. I worked with more deliberation: everything I did was a ritual where the smallest detail took on great significance. My family and friends became even more important than they had previously. I moved about slowly but surely, savoring all aspects of life. I began to realize how precious a gift life is, and I was determined not to lose that gift.

My children noticed the change in me. They noticed that I was quieter, almost distracted. My eldest son, David, asked me what was wrong one day, and I told him I was just worried about the tests I had to take at the hospital. I didn't elaborate, but spoke in generalities, not wanting to disturb him or the others without cause.

Children, though, are acutely aware of their surroundings. They know when something's wrong. My children heard me crying silently by myself. They overheard the many phone calls to family and friends. They eavesdropped while Wayne and I talked about our situation. They were shaken when Wayne would scold them for being noisy and tell them that their mother "had enough to worry about without you guys running around the house like wild Indians."

Others in our family were shaken as well. My mother took it hard, and I'm sure my father did, though he never said so. My sisters and the in-laws were disturbed by the news. But Wayne's mother, Gladys, was most affected.

We had been close since I first met her in my senior year of high school. She was a warmhearted and generous woman and welcomed me into her home. Though she didn't want Wayne and me to marry when we did, at the age of twenty, she immediately made me feel like part of the family. I will always love her for that.

She was hardest hit because in the past sixteen months, cancer had taken away her brother, her brother-in-law, her nephew, and a cousin. She had lost a great deal to the disease and was determined not to let it take another person she loved. She and my mother, along with Wayne, became my strongest supporters.

Two weeks later, Wayne and I went to The Breast Center. The doctors wanted to determine if the area of calcification was in fact cancerous.

They had originally planned to biopsy only the area of calcification; they weren't concerned about the lumps I had discovered. I told them that I wasn't comfortable with that and wanted the lumps examined as well. They agreed and decided to do a needle aspiration to check the lumps. The wheel of calcification could not be checked by the "blind entry" of the needle aspiration and would have to wait for the normal biopsy at a later date.

I was nervous as one of the nurses led me back to an examining room. Wayne held my hand tightly and told me everything would be all right. My surgeon, Dr. Silverstein (whose card I had absently picked out from the stack on the receptionist's desk the day I discovered I had cancer), explained to me what he was going to do.

"It's really pretty simple," he said. "We'll place the hypodermic needle into the area that we want to sample and take out a little bit of tissue. Then we'll examine that and determine what is to be done from the results."

Though he was careful not to hurt me any more than necessary, the process was uncomfortable. Dr. Silverstein probed both areas with the needle until he found the right spot and then removed a small sample from each. After the last bit of tissue was removed, I stood and began to put on my bra. Doctor Silverstein stopped me and told me there was one more thing they had to do.

"It's just standard procedure really. But we have to get a picture of your breasts," he said reassuringly.

He left the room and the technician took the picture. In spite of what the doctor had said, I was not convinced that this was standard procedure. I was chilled to the bone by the thought that the photograph would be used later during the reconstruction of my breast. When she finished taking the Polaroid picture, I dressed quickly and without a word walked down to the consulting room to wait for Dr. Silverstein. Wayne walked behind me lost in his own thoughts.

The doctor joined us in the consultation room and told us that he felt the lumps were benign but that the aspiration would help tell for sure. He said he thought there may be some treatment necessary for the cluster of calcification, but that it may not be too serious.

"I don't want you to worry, Becky. Just go home and try to relax and we'll contact you in a few days about the tests. So far, everything looks under control, but we won't be sure until we get the results from the lab."

2

Suspicion Confirmed

I slept poorly that night. A million thoughts ran through my mind as I tossed and turned in bed. I thought about how healthy I had always been, how everything had always worked out fine in the past. I was trying to be positive, telling myself I could face whatever came my way with courage, but fear crept into my mind.

The next day Dr. Silverstein called.

I was sitting at the kitchen table, having just put my daughter Aimee down for her afternoon nap. I was relaxing for a moment with a glass of iced tea, waiting for the boys to come home from school.

When the phone rang, my heart skipped a beat. I instinctively knew who was calling. I wasn't sure if I wanted to hear what he had to say. I let the phone ring a number of times before I got up and answered it.

"Hello," I said timidly into the mouthpiece.

"Hello, Becky?"

"Yes."

"This is Dr. Silverstein, Becky. We've got the results back from your aspiration."

"What is it, doctor."

"Well, the results are very suspicious. . . ."

My mind froze for a moment, and his words passed over me as if intended for someone else. I stared through the kitchen window without thinking. I could see the trees in our neighbor's yard bending before the wind outside and a jet streak across the gray sky, but everything was silent. I was afraid to ask him what he meant.

" . . . You seem to have some atypical cells," he added.

"What do you mean by that?" I asked in a daze.

"Well, Becky, it just means that we've found something abnormal about the cells in the lumps you discovered. But we really can't tell right now what that is." He paused for a moment. "I wish I could be more specific, but we just don't know right now. The sample we took was too small, and we'll have to do a biopsy to determine if there is a problem or not."

"How serious is it?"

"I don't know, and I don't want to give you any ideas about this unless I'm sure. I can tell you that there's something unusual about both the sites we examined, and, of course, we want to check the area of calcification."

We talked for a while, and then he put me through to the receptionist and I made an appointment for a few days later to have a biopsy of the three areas.

Once again, Wayne was a source of strength for me. When he came home that evening, I wrapped my arms around him and buried my face in his chest. I told him I needed more tests and that things did not look good. He assured me it was not time to worry yet and told me we'd take things one step at a time.

The rest of the family did not know exactly what I was

going through. I told them, of course, that the doctors had found something, but I wasn't specific. I didn't want to tell anyone how serious it was until I was sure one way or the other. There was no reason to worry them unnecessarily. I just told them I needed more tests—they worried enough about that.

I didn't want to worry others, but there was no way I could keep from worrying myself. I discovered the lumps at the end of August and had been struggling with fear and anxiety for weeks. Regardless of how the tests came out, the encounter had already taken its toll.

The three days between the doctor's call and my biopsy crept by like a suspicious cat. If it were possible, I would have slowed time even more. I wanted time to stop. I didn't want to face what I knew was coming.

Once again we drove to The Breast Center in silence. As we drove, I felt a sense of déjà vu come over me. I felt almost as if I were having a familiar and haunting nightmare: a nightmare I could not escape, a nightmare that only occurred under the harsh gaze of reality.

The streets of Van Nuys seemed as familiar as the streets of my hometown. The elevator looked like one I had ridden every day of my life. Walking into The Breast Center felt as normal as walking into the hospital where I worked. The receptionists, the technicians, the patients, were all as familiar as co-workers. I felt as if I had been there a dozen times before. I somehow knew that I would be there many times again.

After a few minutes, a technician called my name. I stood, looked at Wayne for a moment, and followed her back to an examining room. She explained the procedure as we went.

"We'll be taking another mammogram so we can pinpoint the three areas we're going to examine," she said, opening the door to the same examining room I had entered before. "The area of calcification is so small it can not be felt so it's necessary to use a procedure called needle locatization. With this technique long thin wires are inserted into the breast, using mammography to pinpoint the area to be biopsied. The lumps you found are big enough so we don't have to use the wires to find them for the biopsy." I looked at the wires and winced. They seemed as thick as darning needles. I was glad they had to use them for only one area. "Please take off your blouse and bra, Becky, and we'll get started."

It was an uncomfortable process, but not terribly painful. The technician placed my breast in the X-ray machine that had been used on my previous visit, took an X-ray, and then ran the film over to the viewing room for Dr. Gamagami to examine. Soon the doctor came in and injected my breast with Novocain to ease the pain. Then he stuck the wires into my breast at the proper points indicated from the mammogram. Another X-ray was taken. The doctor examined the film, and then adjusted the wires so the area could be pinpointed more precisely.

After the wires were properly placed, the nurses gave me a gown to wear. I was led across the hall to the operating room. The technician told me to lie down on a gurney in the waiting area. The last thing I remember is someone telling me he was putting me under general anesthesia and that when I woke up it would all be over.

When I awoke my breast felt as if it were on fire. My entire chest was wrapped from my armpits to my waist. The wraps were so tight, I had difficulty breathing.

After the biopsy, I was supposed to have a preliminary diagnosis from the center's pathologist. He was not available when I awoke, so Dr. Silverstein talked to me and told me a diagnosis wasn't possible until the tissue was studied. I'd heard that story many times during my years as a nurse and knew that more often than not it meant the worst. I also noticed how quiet everyone was. I knew from experience that when the news was bad, silence prevailed. Still, I thought I would need only a lumpectomy. I didn't realize how advanced the cancer was. With my mind in a whirl, I made an appointment to see the doctor the next day.

I was quiet and pensive when I got home. My chest still burned from the biopsy, and I still had difficulty breathing. I was in a daze, but the residual effects of the anesthesia weren't sufficient to block the thought pounding in my brain that cancer had taken hold of me. I was thankful that my mother and Wayne's mother decided to come and stay with us for a few days. They were a big help, not only by encouraging me, but by doing things around the house until I could get back on my feet. It was hard for me to concentrate enough to take care of my family.

Mom and Gladys cooked, cleaned, and ran errands, but as helpful as they were, they couldn't help with certain things. No one could help me deal with my fear of cancer. I waited anxiously for the phone to ring and for one of my doctors to tell me everything was fine, that I wouldn't have to return to the center. The call never came, though, and the next day we drove to the center under a cloud of doubt to hear the diagnosis.

I was nervous and upset the next morning as we got ready to go to The Breast Center. After breakfast, I was sick to my stomach from worry. I was as quiet as a statue as we drove into Van Nuys once again.

That pensiveness had become part of my personality. I ignored my family and friends and was oblivious of my surroundings. My only concern was the next visit to the doctor's office. When we finally got to The Breast Center, the world began to fall down around me.

We were both led into a consultation room, where we waited only a moment before Dr. Silverstein arrived. As soon as he sat down, I knew I was in trouble. He coughed, cleared his throat, then looked at me with compassionate eyes. "Well, Becky, the news is bad," he said, gently stroking his dark beard. "There's just no way to make it anything else. You have cancer of the breast here, here, and here." He dropped his hand and pointed to his own chest to show me the areas at the top, side, and bottom. "It's kinda' like a ladder, running from the left side of the breast all the way to the top."

The words hit me like a physical blow. For a moment, I didn't believe what he said. But there was no denying it.

I knew breast cancer sometimes spread into the lymph nodes and asked him if mine seemed to be headed that way. He was reluctant to venture a guess, but I pressed him. He finally agreed it was possibility.

"There's about a 20 percent chance that the cancer got into your lymph nodes," he said reluctantly. "That, I'm afraid, would be very bad news indeed," he added with a sigh.

Those words shut the door on any hope I had. I suspected that I would have only about five years to live if the cancer got into my lymph nodes. The fact that there was an 80 percent chance that the lymph nodes would be benign was lost on me. I was convinced I was going to die. I immediately thought of my children and wondered what life would be like for them if I were gone.

He told me I would have to have a mastectomy, the complete removal of the breast. "There's just too much cancer to get away with a lumpectomy, Becky. I'm sorry. During the operation, we'll remove some lymph nodes from your left arm pit and examine them for malignancies. I think there's a good chance that everything will be fine as far as that's concerned, but I suggest you schedule surgery as soon as possible. I don't want to scare you, but this is serious, Becky. Very serious."

I was dumbfounded by what he said. I barely remember Wayne thanking the doctor and leading me out of the consultation room. In the reception area, he scheduled a date for the surgery, which was to be done at the hospital next door. One of the women who worked at the center talked to me briefly and tried to reassure me, but I was in shock and really didn't hear much of what she said. I looked around the waiting room as Wayne finalized the plans. I thought about how smug I had been when I was there for the first time a few weeks before. I don't think I will ever be that smug again as long as I live.

There was no turning back now, no denial. I had to face a serious threat to my life: a threat that was living inside me, growing every day. Once again, I rode home from The Breast Center in a daze.

I couldn't let the fog envelop me, though. When we got home, I had to face the family and come to grips with the wide influence this disease would have.

Before we even got to the front porch, my middle son, Stephen, threw open the front door and came out to see me. He smiled up at me, thinking everything was all right, not knowing the bad news I had just heard.

I hugged him and tears welled up in my eyes. Without a word, I gently ushered him into the house. The other boys were standing around the living-room couch. David, my eldest, just looked at me with a worry-filled face I didn't think a ten-year-old boy could possess. Aaron and Aimee, though concerned, were a little too young really to know what was going on.

"Boys," Wayne said, closing the door. "I want to talk to you about something. Why don't we all go into Mom and Dad's bedroom." He looked tired and worried but showed no panic. I'm sure he was trying to be brave not only for me but for our children and the rest of the family.

As they padded down the hall into the bedroom, Gladys gently grabbed Wayne by the arm. He looked at her questioning eyes and nodded his head. "She's going to have to have a mastectomy—soon."

"You knew all along, didn't you?" she said in a whisper, pain etched on her face.

"No, Mom," Wayne said with a sigh. "I didn't know. I wasn't sure. I had my suspicions, but that's all."

"But why didn't you let us know?" I could tell she was hurt by having been left in the dark.

"We just figured there was no sense worrying everybody until we knew for sure." He patted her on the shoulder and then walked away to tell his boys that their mother was very sick and needed an operation.

Gladys wilted. She sat heavily on the sofa and buried her face in her hands. "Oh, God!" she groaned as she wept. "Not Becky, too!"

My heart ached as I looked at her. I could hardly

imagine the pain she was feeling, after having lost so many loved ones to cancer. I sat down beside her, and my mother sat beside me, and we all wept.

3

A Black Cloud

Because of the bad news, our mothers decided to stay with us for a few more days. We were both glad to have them around: they were good with the kids and quite comforting. I thanked God we had such caring people in our lives.

That afternoon I called my sisters and some of my friends to tell them about my cancer. My sisters were deeply hurt by the news, but like the rest of us, were almost expecting it. They offered to help all they could. I asked them to pray for me. My friends responded the same way, and I told them also I could use their prayers. Everyone was supportive, helpful, and filled with love, but that did little to ease my pain.

After making the calls, I stood in the kitchen and thought about my troubles. I started thinking about how unfair it was. I couldn't believe God wanted my life to end this way. He couldn't want my children to grow up without a mother. From the living room I could hear Gladys and my mom talking. I could hear Wayne gently talking to the boys. I smiled for the first time that day, realizing what support I had in my family, and what a loving man Wayne was.

I began to think about our life together. I began to drift back through the years ... back to high school when we first met.

It sounds corny, but Wayne and I had the type of romance that was custom-made for teen novels. He was a handsome athlete and scholar. I was a cheerleader who had numerous friends, good grades, and an eye for the future. We were full of life and deeply in love.

We had known each other since we were sophomores at Ramona High School in Riverside, California. I was a "B" cheerleader, and Wayne was a star on the "B" football team. I thought he was cute and had my eye on him from the first day I saw him on the practice field, but he never paid much attention to me. He later claimed it was because all the other boys were hanging around, and he couldn't get a word in edgewise. I still think he was more interested in his grades and sports than he was in girls.

When we were seniors, Wayne began to take a little more interest in girls. Luckily, his interest focused on me. It came at a good time for the two of us. The boy I had been unenthusiastically dating was away at college. Perhaps Wayne figured he then had a green light.

We didn't have a real "date" for quite a while. We always did things with a few friends or in a group. We did what other teenagers were doing that typically warm fall of 1968. We ate pizza at the local hangout, participated in school activities, and occasionally went to parties.

Sometimes we got a little crazy. While we were out with some friends one Saturday night, Wayne decided to put some excitement into the evening. He drove his dad's 1965

Malibu out into the orange groves to an old railroad crossing. He drove the car onto the tracks and with the tires
hugging the tops of the rails, rolled slowly into the night
with the lights out. We laughed and giggled and screamed,
enjoying the sheer lunacy of it all, oblivious to the danger.
The fun lasted until the tires slipped off the tracks. Then
we pounded across the railroad ties until we reached the
next crossing. We felt wild and free, doing something deli-
cious, naughty, and forbidden. We were kids.

By the time we graduated, we knew we wanted to spend
the rest of our lives together. Wayne went to the University
of California at Riverside, and I took nursing courses at
Riverside City College. At the time, I wasn't all that
interested in nursing. All I wanted was to get a good job so
that after Wayne and I got married I could work while he
finished his education. Later, though, I fell in love with the
profession.

Two years after high school, we were married. Those
were lean times, but they were good times for us. Wayne
attended the university on an athletic scholarship. We both
worked part-time, and Wayne's parents paid for his books.
We lived in subsidized housing for $95.31 a month, includ-
ing utilities. The day we got married, we had $500 to our
name.

By the time Wayne was a senior, I had my nursing
credential and was working full-time. Money was no
longer a problem. Life was good.

Two years later, our lives improved even more. We were
expecting our first child in December, and we were
concerned about how we were going to raise him. I ran
into an old friend who had been really wild in high school,
and she told me how Christ had changed her life. She

invited us to Easter services with her. Since we had no plans, we decided to go. We found an entire world we had never known existed. We met a new breed of people: men and women whom we could befriend easily and grow close to in a very short while. Our new friends glowed with tranquillity, and they cared about others. Unlike so many couples we knew, they could have fun without going to wild parties, or drinking, or carrying on like fools. They had something really special, and we knew that was what we wanted in our lives.

Though we had a happy marriage, we both knew something was missing—that there was a void in our lives. We went to church, when it was convenient, and began to consider the Christian faith. Soon we were examining the life of Christ and wondering if he would fit into our lives. We read and researched to determine if we wanted to follow Christian doctrine. Finally, in my last month of pregnancy, we became Christians. We found what was missing in our lives.

In January of 1976 our first son, David, was born. Two years later Stephen was born, and Wayne received his doctorate in biochemistry. He got a grant to do postdoctoral research for the National Institute of Health and Medical Research in France. So, we loaded up the family and moved to a country as alien to us as the rocky face of the moon.

We spent a year in France and were very glad to come home. Wayne decided not to stay in the academic world. Instead, he accepted a position as a research scientist with a medical laboratory in Van Nuys. To celebrate, we had our third son, Aaron.

We finally completed our family when Aimee was born

in May of 1983. I had prayed for a little girl and now my prayers were answered. Her birth was one of the highlights of my life.

In the meantime, Wayne slowly began moving his way up the corporate ladder. After a few years, he was transferred to San Francisco to take over as site director for his company's two laboratories. We stayed in the Bay Area until Wayne's transfer back to Los Angeles almost two years later.

We were not altogether happy with the transfer. We had made a home in northern California. It was cleaner, less crowded than the Los Angeles area, and a better place to raise our four children. Wayne briefly thought about striking out on his own, but he stayed with the company and we reluctantly moved back in February of 1986. Seven months later, the tumor was discovered on my breast.

I really don't think I would be alive today if we had not moved back to southern California. To my knowledge, there is no facility in the Bay Area like The Breast Center. It's one of the most prestigious facilities of its type in the country. Most of our family lived in southern California as well, and that contributed to my recovery almost as much as the medical attention I received.

Wayne and I feel it was God's hand that directed us back to our roots. We also feel God led us to the gynecologist who recommended The Breast Center. It was no coincidence that the facility was just two miles from Wayne's laboratory and he could visit me without missing much work. Of course, all of that was not so apparent when I was in the middle of my crisis.

It certainly wasn't apparent the day I was told I must have a mastectomy. I was deeply troubled by the news, but not because I was afraid to lose my breast. For some reason, that really didn't bother me. Most women fear disfigurment; the fear of dying was what caused me the most grief.

The day my world came crumbling down, I thought constantly about my family and my death. I didn't want my children to be left without a mother, or Wayne to be left without a wife. For a while, I even thought about what would happen if I died. I wondered what kind of life my children would have without me there to help them. I wondered what kind of life Wayne would build for himself. I wondered if he would remarry, and if he did, if his new wife would be good to my children. I was afraid death was just biding its time, waiting for me. I wondered how I would die and hoped it be a quick death, not a lingering slide into oblivion. I didn't want my children to remember me as a wasted vestige of what I had been.

The boys stayed outside that day and generously allowed Aimee to play with them. Wayne and I moved around the house as quietly as cats, doing little things to keep ourselves busy. We were trying not to think about the obvious, but every time we looked at each other I burst into tears. A black cloud had descended on the Wecksler family. We could only pray that it wouldn't stay.

4

Prayers of Faith

It's been said thousands of times, and I believe it: God works in strange ways. For that reason, to a Christian there is no such thing as coincidence. Everything is part of God's plan. When Pastor Jim Frost called me only hours after I had been told I needed a mastectomy, God's plan was continuing. Of course, I didn't see it at the time.

Jim had heard about my problem from a friend of his. It seems his friend's wife had talked to my sister-in-law, Charlotte, about what we had been going through. The message was passed along to Jim.

We really didn't talk much that first night he called. He just said that he heard we had no permanent support group or church and asked if we needed people with whom to pray. I told him we did, and he agreed to visit the next Saturday and pray with us.

I felt a little better when I hung up the phone. It wasn't because of what Jim had said, but because I knew inside that God had been working in my life and I had not been aware enough to notice. Wayne and I talked about it that night and we both felt that in our self-concern, we had put

God on the back burner. Neither one of us had given our-selves fully to God since the cancer became apparent weeks before. Though we prayed often, we weren't quite ready to put it all in God's hands. I guess we were trying to handle it on our own. I was to learn later that it just couldn't be done. I needed God to take over my burden.

We tried our best to live life in a normal way, but it wasn't easy. Wayne went to work and continued with his night classes at UCLA. He was well into the master's program there, and we both felt it would be foolish for him to quit. It was not only important for our future and im-portant for us to plan the future, it also kept his mind off our troubles. Since I was working only part-time at the hos-pital, I felt it would not be fair for me to go back to work for a short time only to quit again when I had to have the operation. The staff was helpful, and I was told my job would be waiting for me when I returned.

We went through the next few days trying to maintain a sense of normality. The children went about their usual activities, though a little more quietly, and Wayne and I did the same. We fretted, worried, and prayed, hoping for the best.

By that Saturday, we both felt as if we needed some Christian fellowship. The day was a normally hectic one, and by the time we put the children to bed, we were tired but excited about having someone to pray with. Shortly after the kids were tucked away, Jim Frost and his wife, Emily, came to the door with their friends, Alan and Deb-bie Burnett.

We served them coffee and cookies, and we all sat in our living room and talked. It was mainly small talk at first, just to get to know each other. Gradually we began to talk about my breast cancer and how God could work with us if we let him.

Jim, who was pastor of a small church in Valencia, asked us if we'd like to read James 5:13, referring to God's healing powers. We all agreed.

"And the prayer of faith shall save the sick," he said, continuing to read from the New Testament as the rest of us silently read along with him. "And the Lord shall raise him up; and if he have committed sins, they shall be forgiven him. Confess your faults one to another, and pray one for another, that ye may be healed" (KJV). He stopped reading and looked at me. "That's what we're here for tonight, Becky. We're here to pray with you and ask God to work in your life and help you over these troubled times."

I began to think about what he had said. I knew that according to the Scriptures, unconfessed sin would hinder God's ability to work in my life. I tried to think of what I had held back. I didn't know what it could be.

"Becky, God's only request is that we become transparent before him in order to receive his blessing of healing. If there's anything you haven't given to the Lord, just say so now. Let God see your sins or tell him about something you haven't yet let go of."

Suddenly, I knew what it was God wanted from me. For years I had held inside a deep resentment for my alcoholic father. Though I had prayed for him and forgiven him in my words, I had never really forgiven him in my heart. I had never really let go of the pain and anger I'd felt since early childhood when I needed him and he was never available. I was also angry that he had not even expressed his concern over my present illness.

"There's one thing," I said to Jim, with tears beginning to well up in my eyes. "It's my father." I told the group about his alcoholism and told them about how he had ignored my disease and had offered no comfort. I told them he even seemed to resent my mother spending so much time with me.

Jim looked at me with moist eyes. "Let us pray," he said. We were silent for a moment, in our own way asking God to help me. Then Jim told me to repeat his prayer. "Becky, repeat after me: Lord, you know my father has hurt me...."

"Lord, you know my father has hurt me...."

"You know I've tried to forgive him in the past but failed."

"You know I've tried to forgive him in the past but failed."

"If I could not forgive him before, I forgive him now. In Jesus' name, Amen."

I finished the prayer and tears were flowing down my cheeks. I looked over at Wayne, and he was also crying. The others had moist eyes as well.

Jim then anointed my forehead with oil and asked the Holy Spirit to come into my body and heal me of the cancer that was destroying my life. He also asked God to give Wayne the strength to support me through my troubles.

We prayed a while longer and then the others decided to leave. On the way out the door, Jim asked me if I had felt God move within me. I told him I felt a certain peace that I always feel when I pray but nothing like a lightning bolt or sudden insight. He just nodded. Jim suggested we have another prayer session before the operation, and I agreed.

As Wayne and I prepared for bed, I felt a little touch of calm but no dramatic change. I still puzzled over what Jim had been driving at but dismissed it. A few days later, I had my first real sign that God was working in my life. It was only a beginning.

5

A Daze of Consultations

When I had talked to Dr. Silverstein the day he gave me the bad news, he suggested I get a second opinion. He also wanted Wayne and me to come back to discuss the surgery and reconstruction.

I got the second opinion soon after our prayer session with Jim Frost. It substantiated what the doctors at The Breast Center had told me. I never thought it would be anything different. The second doctor suggested I had a 40 percent chance the cancer was in my lymph nodes and that I might consider having both breasts removed. It was hardly a cheerful prognosis.

Wayne and I, along with Mom and Gladys, went back to the center a couple days after I got the second opinion. We were scheduled to talk to Dr. Hoffman, the center's psychiatrist. Then we were to meet with Dr. Silverstein and other members of the staff.

The first consultation and the ones that followed were a blur. I couldn't concentrate on what was said, because every time I returned to The Breast Center the word CANCER echoed in my mind. I do remember talking to the psychiatrist that first time, though, and feeling a great deal of comfort at what he said.

During our conversation with Dr. Hoffman, Wayne finally broke down and cried. He had been so strong for so long, but I was pleased that he finally showed his emotion. It gave him a release from all the feelings he had bottled up. It also gave me an opportunity to comfort him, an opportunity that I relished. Dr. Hoffman told me that most women normally fit the role of comforter. Therefore, they don't feel right when they need to be comforted. He said I should allow others to care for me: words that I remembered all through the ordeal. He also talked to my mother and mother-in-law that day. He told them how I would react to the surgery and what they could do to help me through the rough days ahead. I never went back to talk to the psychiatrist, but it was comforting to talk to him that one time. It was reassuring to know that he'd be there if I needed him.

Later, we met with Dr. Silverstein and the other members of the team at The Breast Center. We met the oncologist, Dr. James Waisman; the plastic surgeon, Dr. Handel; and the patient educator, Ellen Waisman, Dr. Waisman's sister. It was Ellen who had comforted me the day I received the bad news. She was to continue to give me courage throughout the ordeal.

Once again we were led back to a consultation room. Once again experts were going to give me information about the upcoming ordeal. As we talked, the word CANCER filled my thoughts.

"I'm glad you could make it today," Dr. Silverstein said, gesturing for us to sit down. "I think it's very important for us to talk things over, to discuss what's going to happen, and your feelings about that. Whenever we deal with cancer, we like to take a holistic approach, if you will. In other words, your feelings, your attitude, and your ability to fight the disease are all part of the process."

Wayne and I both nodded our heads in agreement. We had discussed the problem, and had come to the conclusion that I could fight it. My attitude would be an important tool in the battle.

"Your overall attitude is very important," Dr. Silverstein continued, as if reading my mind. "It seems to us that you've come to grips with your situation quickly. In other words, you're not denying you have the disease—which is common."

"I guess there's no sense denying it," I said.

He shook his head. "No. There's not."

We sat quietly for a moment. "There's another thing I want you both to know. A number of patients get the notion that they have somehow brought this on themselves. But there is no evidence that personality has anything to do with getting cancer. Certain personalities may be more susceptible to it, but we don't really know. Nobody knows. Some researchers feel there is a connection, others don't. One thing that seems certain to everyone is that personality has a lot to do with recovery."

"You mean having a positive attitude?" I asked.

"Yes. That, and how you feel about the disease. It seems you have faced it, and reconciled yourself to it, and that's good. You're in touch with your feelings. You have no—oh, confusion, I guess—about the cancer. I think with an aggressive treatment and your attitude, we'll be able to whip this, and you'll leave it behind. That's healthy."

"That's right," Ellen said. "Some patients never come to

grips with cancer, and recovery is that much more difficult because of it."

Dr. Silverstein sat forward and then cleared his throat. "What we try to do here is let the patient know just what's going on. We feel that brings better results." He adjusted his glasses and then ran his hand through his hair. "What I'd like to do is just sort of walk through the surgery with you, so you know what to expect. First of all, when you go into the hospital, we'll do a bone scan. As you know, we inject a minute amount of radioactive material into the vein and that is carried throughout the body by the blood. We can then tell by X-ray if any of the bones, or liver, have been affected by the disease."

I nodded my head and nervously twisted my hands in my lap. I felt strange having someone discuss me in such a clinical way. Though as a nurse I had done so many times about patients, it was strange to have the tables turned.

"What we're suggesting is a modified radical mastectomy. In the old days they'd take the breast and a great deal of underlying muscle tissue, but that's rarely done anymore. We've found it's not worth the extra trauma for the minute chance that the cancer has spread into the muscle. The modified is a much less debilitating operation. We'll also be removing some of the lymph nodes in your left armpit. That's done so we can see if they're cancerous or not."

I told him what the other doctor had told me about the removal of both breasts.

"Well, that's why we have you get a second opinion. That way you have options. If you feel confident in that diagnosis, I'd be wrong to try and talk you out of it. We feel that the removal of both breasts is unnecessary. As to the chances of your getting lymph cancer, the difference between 20 and 40 is just a matter of opinion, really. I don't think the difference should worry you."

Dr. Handel explained the various types of reconstructive surgery following the removal of the breast. I wasn't that concerned about the reconstruction; I mainly wanted to save my life. I didn't want to look like a "freak," of course, but I wasn't greatly concerned with how the reconstruction was done. I wanted to be symmetrical and continue my active life. Otherwise, it didn't matter.

He explained how tissue from the abdomen or the back can be transplanted to the breast, and he also told me about an implant. "The first two have the advantage of using your own tissue and ending up with a more natural-looking breast," he said. I told him I thought the implant might be the least damaging of the procedures.

"That's right," Dr. Handel said. "It doesn't involve any taking of tissue, so therefore it is less traumatic. I think that may be the procedure for you, but of course, you'll have to decide. We're not going to try and talk you into doing anything you're not comfortable with."

"The process begins after surgery when we place a balloon-type device under the skin where the breast was. This tissue-expander is injected with a saline solution every week or so to expand the skin. Once the skin is stretched, a prosthesis can be placed under the skin, and a natural-like breast may be formed."

"Won't that make it more difficult for new tumors to be detected?" I asked.

"There doesn't seem to be much problem detecting new tumors behind or around an implant," he added. "If you want, we can discuss this in more detail when you come in next week to see our video on breast reconstruction."

Dr. Waisman nodded and said, "After surgery, chemotherapy is sometimes called for. But that may not be necessary, so we don't need to really discuss it now. I should say that it is an excellent preventive procedure. We believe in aggressively treating cancer, and that sometimes includes chemotherapy. If tests indicate that it's needed, we'll recommend that you do it."

I absently nodded my head. Everything was coming at me so fast I could hardly think. I was facing a major surgery and all these people were telling me about reconstruction, chemotherapy, and other problems I couldn't think about at the time. My face must have given away my feelings, because Ellen looked at me with a wry grin.

"I know we're covering a lot of territory, Becky," she said, "but we think it's important that you know what's in store for you and deal with it as a whole."

Dr. Silverstein and the others stood. "I think I've covered about all I need to," he said. "Maybe it would be better, Becky, if you and Ellen just talked things over. I think you'll find her both knowledgeable and understanding," he smiled.

He turned to Wayne and asked him to step outside with him and doctors Handel and Waisman. They left and gently closed the door. For some reason I felt relieved. It would be nice to sit and talk with another woman about all I was going through.

We talked for a while, with Ellen just comforting me and giving me encouragement. When we ended the conversation she told me a little more about the various procedures for the mastectomy and reconstruction. She said the final choice was mine on what procedure to follow, but that the doctors come to their conclusions based on a great deal of experience and knowledge. I thanked her and left the consulting room feeling good about the fact that the doctors wanted me to be an integral part of the decision-making process.

6

Gathering Strength

I felt much better after we discussed my surgery and recovery with the staff at The Breast Center. I was especially comforted by Ellen, but I still had a great deal of fear. I still did not put my life completely in God's hands. Things soon started to happen that convinced me to do so.

When we left The Breast Center, we reaffirmed the fact that the surgery would be set for the following Tuesday. I was told to come into The Valley Medical Center next door a day early for some tests and to prepare for surgery. Of course, the next few days would be filled with tension, but with a little help from my sister, I managed to find a way to deal with that.

I invited Susan to come to The Breast Center with me and view the videotape about the reconstruction. We laughed about picking the "perfect pair" for me and acted about as mature as a couple of teenagers. Neither of us felt silly, though. It was important for me to keep my sense of humor, or I would collapse under the weight of my problems.

But I couldn't act goofy all the time. I had to get on with

my life as well as I could. I didn't realize that just by living my life as normally as possible, I would get some lessons on how to deal with my problem.

Weeks before I found out about the cancer, we had planned to take a trip to Marineland with the Tiger Cubs, a boy-scout-like group my boys belonged to. The date was the Sunday before I was scheduled to go into the hospital.

I had mixed feelings about going. I thought it was silly and frivolous to be doing something "fun" when my life was in such danger. On the other hand, it seemed like the perfect way to get my mind off my troubles. After discussing it with Wayne, I decided it would be best to go ahead and make the trip. It was one of the best decisions of my life.

With high hopes for a good day, we piled the kids into the car that Sunday morning. The boys, naturally, were excited and therefore a handful. I tried to ignore their squabbling and silliness, figuring they, too, had been under pressure and needed some fun. We met the other parents at a local McDonald's and then drove in a caravan to Marineland.

Saugus' Frontier Days parade was also planned for that morning. As we drove toward the freeway the traffic was slowed to a crawl because the main street was being roped off for the parade. I was daydreaming as we rolled along. In spite of myself, I was thinking about the surgery and staring out the windshield. Suddenly, out of the corner of my eye, I noticed something move in the car next to us. I had a feeling something odd was happening. My heart skipped a beat when I realized the man driving the car was having some type of seizure.

Time crawled. The scene passed before my eyes like a

movie in slow motion. The man sat behind the wheel shaking uncontrollably, struggling for his breath. He wasn't even looking at the road, and his late-model sedan was rolling out of control next to us.

"Wayne, stop!" I shouted, opening the car door as my startled husband slammed on the brakes. "I think he's having a heart attack," I explained, as I ran toward the man's car. His sedan angled away from us and then started slowly drifting back into our lane. I opened the door and steered the slow-moving car over the right-hand curb almost into a brick wall. I turned off the engine and undid the man's seat belt as he continued to struggle uncomprehendingly.

I laid him on the ground next to the car. I loosened his tie and unbuttoned his shirt so I could feel for his carotid pulse in his neck. Before I had a chance to do anything else, two paramedics came up beside me and knelt next to the man. As soon as I saw he was in good hands, I stood up and went back to our car, which by now was blocking traffic.

My kids cheered me when I got back in and asked me if the man was dead. I told them I thought he would be fine. Wayne said I looked like Annie Oakley bulldogging the car to a stop. We laughed, flushed with excitement.

As we drove, I began thinking about how precious life was. I began thinking that it wasn't just luck that put me next to that man. I felt God's hand working in my life and figured if God was going to put me in a position to save someone's life, he probably wasn't going to end mine. I wasn't sure, of course, but the thought made me feel better than I had in a long time.

We had a wonderful time at Marineland. I was glad we took the children, whose usual antics while in public pleased me rather than drove me to madness. I was also thankful for the opportunity to do what I had done for the man.

When we got home that evening, we were all feeling really good for the first time in weeks. The children had a wonderful time and were pleased that they made it through a day without getting yelled at. Wayne was happy because he noticed that I was feeling better.

Wayne decided to make dinner for us that evening.

"I want you to appreciate your hospital food, Beck," he said jokingly. "The best way to do that, is to have something really bad to compare it to."

I smiled at him and sat down at the kitchen table to look through the previous day's mail. To my surprise, I found a letter from my father.

My hands shook a little as I opened it. I had not talked much to my father since all this started, and he had never offered me any compassion. I guess I was a little stunned by the letter. I was certainly curious about what he had to say.

The stationery made me chuckle. It had an angel jumping up in front of a basketball net, slamming the ball through the hoop. I couldn't figure out exactly what was meant by that, but it was cute. The letter read:

> Dear Becky,
>   This is not the first crisis we've had but probably the greatest. The first was your "blanket" which I had to take away from you. The second was your teeth when you could eat popcorn out of a coke bottle and you overcame that. From that time forward I knew you could do anything you set your mind to do.
>   You became a leader of people from sophomore princess to basketball sweetheart.

You reached your goal, with your marriage and your children. They have become leaders too.

No matter how great the crisis is, Becky, you can conquer it.

All love, Dad

P.S.: One thing I am not sure you ever took care of was the housework the judge ordered you to do after the warning you received for riding double on the motorcycle.

Tears filled my eyes as I read the letter. I laughed at the part about the Coke bottle and its reference to my buck teeth as a kid. I also laughed at the part about the judge who gave me a stern warning about riding a motorcycle illegally.

Wayne looked over at me and noticed my tears and laughter. "You okay?" he asked, standing in front of the oven with an apron around his waist.

"It's a letter from my dad. It's the first indication he's ever given me that he even cared about my condition." I began to read the letter again.

"Maybe the Lord gave him a little nudge," Wayne said. "Can I see?"

I read it a second time and handed it to him. He read it, and his eyes began to shine. "Wow! That's really nice of him, Beck."

I was convinced that God had touched my father. I just knew he had heard my prayers and now his heavenly hand was working in my life. I felt a warm glow spread through my body. For the first time in weeks, I felt I might have a future.

After dinner I called Pastor Frost. He was excited by the news of the letter and asked if he and his wife could come over to pray with us. Wayne and I both felt that would be fine, and we spent most of the evening in prayer and fellowship.

After they left I felt good about my chances. Wayne and I went to bed, and he comforted me and told me that everything would be all right. He told me he thought God was working on our problem, and that it would work out the way he wanted it to.

In spite of his warm reassurances, I was still afraid. Wayne went to sleep after a while, but I just tossed and turned, unsure of the operation, afraid of all the pain I would have to endure, unconvinced that God was really working with me.

I lay awake for hours, getting less and less confident as time passed. I told myself to sleep, that I needed all the energy I could muster, but I still could not relax. I got up to take a sleeping pill, which I had been doing on occasion lately. Then tried to get back to sleep, but I could not quiet my mind. Finally, at 4:00 a.m., I got up, padded down the hallway, and went out into the backyard.

I sat on a patio chair in the pitch-black night and wept. I felt so lonely and depressed, so fearful of death. I began to pray as I never had before.

"I need your strength. I need your help, Lord," I whispered. "I've never faced anything like this. I've never had to face something I couldn't control or overcome. I've always been able to work a little harder, save a little more, study a little longer, and get over the problem facing me, but not now. This is way too big, Lord. I'm helpless, Lord. Every time I see a doctor, he tells me something worse. I feel like I'm alone, like I'm a little girl again. Like I'm falling down a deep, dark well."

Tears rolled down my cheeks and onto the collar of my

robe. "Please let me know you're with me, Lord. I need to know that you are the one in control of my life. I need to know that this will work out the way you want it to."

I began to think about Jesus, and what it must have been like to suffer so at Calvary. I thought about how he had carried the sins of the world to the cross with him. I asked God to give me the strength that Christ showed. I asked God to take the fear of death away from me. "I want to live, Lord. I want to raise my children and love my husband. I want to do your work. Please take this burden from my shoulders. If you're there, please hear my prayers."

Suddenly, a cool breeze blew out of the still night. It caressed my face and soothed the fires in my mind. Calm came over me, and I heard a gentle voice talking to me as if it whispered from across an empty room.

The voice assured me that I would live. It told me I was in God's hands. It told me to trust in God and tell others that my faith in God would see me through. The voice said I must step out in faith. It said the next few months would be very difficult for me, but that I would live.

With a buoyant heart and a light step, I went back into the house. I glanced at the clock on the kitchen wall and noticed that I had been outside for thirty minutes. It seemed like only five.

I walked down the hallway past the children's bedrooms. I stopped outside the door and listened to their rhythmic breathing. My heart ached in love for them. For a moment, I wanted one of them to cry out so I could go inside and be a comfort. I remembered how much love they had given me, and felt ashamed of all the times I had resented cleaning up after them, or dealing with their squabbles. I thought about what their young lives would be like without a mother and thanked God that they wouldn't find out for a long time.

When I came back to our bedroom, Wayne woke up.

"What time is it?"

"About four-thirty."

"You okay?"

"I'm fine, honey. Everything is just fine. I'm not going to die."

I told him what happened and he cried. "It's just like the poem 'Footprints.' I feel that God is going to carry me through all this and everything is going to be just fine."

We held each other for a long time before falling asleep, knowing just how much we meant to each other.

7

Trauma and Trust

The next morning I checked into the hospital for the bone scan and other tests. I was to stay in the hospital overnight and have the surgery the next morning. Nothing seemed to phase me that day. I was free of fear and doubt for the first time in weeks. I was confident and totally unconcerned about what was going to happen. I was in God's hands.

After checking me in, Wayne went to work. I read from the Bible and listened to Christian tapes on a small portable tape player that I brought with me. Though I was alone, I didn't feel lonely at all. A negative thought never entered my mind. It was almost as if I were on vacation. I knew God was with me.

The Christian songs spoke of trust in God, and as I lay in bed, I knew just what they were talking about. I trusted in God. Only he could have given me the peace that I felt. Only a power greater than man could have made me feel so at ease the day before my surgery.

After a while, I began to read a Christian book my sister Susan had given me. When I opened the book, a bookmark fell out with the poem "Footprints" on it. Wayne and I had talked about the poem the night before, but we couldn't find a copy of it. As I began to read it I realized that this was just another sign that God was working in my life.

The poem is an allegory of our walk with God. In it, a man is shown a stretch of beach where there are two sets of footprints. One pair belongs to the man, the other to God. At one point along the beach, the man sees that there is only one set of footprints. He asked God why He left him alone during that period, and God tells him that when he sees only one set of footprints on the beach, he should know that those were the times God carried him.

Dr. Silverstein, Dr. Waisman, and the plastic surgeon, Dr. Handel, all came in that afternoon to talk over the next day's surgery. I told them I had studied the different procedures, and that I agreed with their opinions. I would go with the modified radical and would have the tissue expander put in during the mastectomy. Dr. Handel told me that I made a wise choice because he didn't think I had enough tissue around my abdomen to use in the other type of reconstruction.

Dr. Waisman told me I seemed to be taking everything well, and I just smiled at him and told him God was on my side. He said the results from the tests were back, and that they looked good. The hormone receptor levels in my tumor were high, which meant the tumor was "mature" and slow-growing. That meant I was a good candidate for recovery. He also said the bone scan was clear and there was no evidence that the cancer had spread to other organs. They would take out some lymph nodes during surgery, he added, to make sure they weren't cancerous.

When they left, I felt even better. They had given me the first good news in a long time. That came less than a day after I had let God control my destiny.

That evening my mother and Gladys came to visit. I told them what had happened and assured them I was going to be just fine. In a little while, we were joined by Wayne and my sisters Susan and Cheryl and my sister-in-law Charlotte. We decided to go out and "celebrate." I got a hospital pass for the evening and went out to dinner with my family.

It's hard to believe how much fun we had. My little sister, Susan, and I made faces at each other. We all told jokes, Wayne even felt some relief from the pressure he had been under and laughed a great deal. My mom and Gladys thought we were a little crazy to be acting that way the day before surgery, but they certainly enjoyed it.

When we got back to the hospital that night, the staff was amazed at our "party" attitude. We were still laughing and joking and goofing around. They could not understand how my family and I could act that way when I was facing such an ordeal the next day, but we didn't care. By that time all of us were confident that everything would be just fine.

Everyone slept in a nearby hotel that night, except for Wayne, who stayed with me. Everybody wanted to be with me as soon as they could the next morning. I thanked God for the love of my family and especially for the love of my husband, whose support for the fifteen years we'd been married was unbelievable.

I felt as if morning would never come. I lay awake all night, thinking about the surgery. I pictured the tube being put down my throat and the anesthesiologist putting me under. I thought about having my breast taken off. I thought about the pain that would be involved.

When the sun finally came up, I was relieved that it would soon be over with. Shortly after sunrise, I went into the hallway so I wouldn't disturb my sleeping husband and prayed. I asked God to make sure the surgery team worked competently. When I went back inside, Wayne was awake. After a while the family arrived, and we talked until it came time for the ride to surgery.

A nurse and an aide came in to put me on the gurney. They had a problem with the bed, though, and couldn't figure out how to drop it down to the proper level. After fiddling with the bed for a while and flopping me all around trying to get me onto the gurney, I got off the bed and hopped onto it like a comic high jumper.

"We got to get this show on the road," I said, settling myself for the ride.

"You must be pretty nervous, honey," the nurse said, joining the laughter. "I've never seen anybody do that."

I must admit I was nervous. I knew what could go wrong in surgery and hoped the surgery team was highly skilled and very competent. In spite of the presence of my family and my faith in God, I began to weep as they wheeled me into the operating room. I was afraid of the pain I would soon be feeling. For the first time I was concerned about my disfigurment.

The anesthesiologist quickly medicated me, and the last thing I remembered were the bright lights above the operating table. Everything from that point on was a fog. The next thing I remembered was waking up many hours later in my hospital room.

My head ached, and I felt disoriented. My arm tingled

as if it were asleep, and my left wrist ached. These pains were much worse than the pain in my chest.

I was told my arm had been in an awkward position during surgery and that the pain would subside. They said the pain in my wrist was normal after such an operation. They also assured me my disorientation would not last.

After I awoke, Wayne massaged my wrist for five hours. Though I felt terrible, I knew things would only get better. I was relieved to have the ordeal over and hopeful that all would now be well.

Wayne stayed with me that night and the next twenty-four hours, during which I was sedated. The next morning we waited for Dr. Waisman to arrive and tell us the results of the biopsy of the lymph nodes. He was scheduled to arrive at noon and we talked calmly as the morning passed, having faith that all would be well. After a while, though, Wayne began to pace back and forth like a caged animal. I noticed the time and realized Dr. Waisman was late. I became anxious myself. Perhaps the biopsy was positive. Perhaps Dr. Waisman was at this very moment trying to find the courage to tell me the cancer had spread.

He finally arrived, and Wayne and I stared intently as he greeted us. When he told me the lymph nodes were not cancerous, I breathed a heavy sigh of relief and thanked God for my health. The doctor felt chemotherapy would be vital for my recovery. He said the size of the removed tumor and my relative youth indicated that I should make sure all the precautions were taken.

"In older patients who have smaller, slow-growing tumors, we often don't recommend chemotherapy," he said, standing next to my bed. "But because you're in your mid-thirties, and the tumor was large, I think it would be wise.

"How bad is it?" I asked, concerned that the drug therapy would be a worse ordeal than what I had already gone through.

"Well, Becky, some patients get very sick, but most of them do just fine. I've found that most of my patients have little problem with chemotherapy. In your case we'll be using small dosages because we found no cancer in the lymph nodes. We'll be using cytoxan, 5 fluorouracil, methotrexate, maybe others. We'll see how you do with one series and then go from there. I think it's vitally important for you to go through with it."

I had mixed feelings about the chemotherapy. I knew it would be a safety measure for me, but I felt that the operation had been a success, and that I should not take a chance on going through another ordeal if I was going to be fine. I figured God had seen me through the surgery, all the cancer was taken from my body, and any other treatment was unnecessary. I was about to say something to Dr. Waisman about my misgivings when Dr. Silverstein came in.

We talked for a moment about the surgery, and he also recommended chemotherapy. He then asked me if I would do him a favor. As with most people, I agreed before I knew what he wanted.

"Sure, Dr. Silverstein. What can I do?"

"Well, Becky. A nurse that I know has been diagnosed as having breast cancer. She's pretty shaken by it, and I thought since you've handled all this so well, you could talk to her."

I was flattered that he thought I had handled my troubles so well. I said I was willing to help. It would do me good to talk to someone in the same situation I was in. It would also give me a chance to witness about God's power.

"I'd love to. When do you want me to see her?"

"Well." He smiled. "We'll give you a day or so to gather your strength. How about Friday? That's the day you check out, isn't it?"

"Friday would be fine," I said.

"Good." He smiled again and told me I was really doing well. Dr. Waisman again assured me chemotherapy would be best for me. I think he saw the reluctance in my face. Then they both left, saying they were pleased with everything so far.

My time in the hospital went by quickly. My family was in and out daily. I felt stronger and stronger every day. I felt as if everything was going to work out.

A few days before I checked out of the hospital, I was visited by a woman from Reach For Recovery, a support group for breast cancer patients. She was helpful and considerate, and I think a little surprised that I needed so little comforting from her. She told me about her chemotherapy and how rough it was. She also told me she lost all her hair, but that it grew back. I think the idea of losing my hair startled me more than losing my breast. Before she left, she gave me a pad for the left side of my bra so I looked symmetrical after discharge.

When I checked out of the hospital, I went next door to The Breast Center and saw the woman who was going to have a mastectomy. It was eerie, sitting in a consultation room at the center, talking to someone else about her breast cancer, but I was glad I could help. I felt God had already begun to use me to help others, and that pleased me.

I felt warmth and love for the woman the moment I set eyes on her frightened face. I hugged her when we met and told her I felt all would go well.

"You're in good hands," I said. "I just had my operation, and everything is fine. I still have my drain in and will for a while, I guess. I think once you come to grips with the surgery and its necessity, you've won half the battle."

She was upset, of course, but she handled it all quite well. She said the news had been bad. "You're the first ray of hope I've had." I got goose bumps when she said that. It seemed at least some good could come from my surgery. We were both nurses and had the exact diagnosis with opposite breasts. Later I visited her in the hospital and continued to see her during her recovery.

My mom and Gladys stayed with us for a week after I got home from the hospital. They did housework and helped with the kids, refusing to let me do anything. I loved having their help and appreciated all that they did, but I was almost glad when they left. That would give me an opportunity to get back on schedule.

I began doing my chores, washing, vacuuming, and scrubbing floors, in spite of my bandages and the recent surgery. After a few days, the left side of my chest began to swell. Worried, I went back to The Breast Center.

Dr. Handel took one look at the wound and said, "What in the world have you been doing?"

"Well, I felt pretty good. I thought I'd do some work around the house."

"What kind of work?"

"Washing, cleaning, just housework."

"Look, Becky, I don't want you doing any of that, you hear? You go home and take it easy. You're not a linebacker, you know." When he redid my bandages he wrapped my arm to my side so I couldn't work. He also decided that since I was there he might as well put in some saline solution for the expander in my chest.

"It'll save you a trip. And I don't expect to see you until you need another dose of saline, all right?"

"Becky," he said as I was about to leave the examining room, "I'm serious. You take it slow. You've gone through a lot, and you can't just jump back into things even if you feel fine."

I told him I would and kept my word. For the next few weeks I moved slowly and let things slide a little. My chest swelled under my arm again, but they wouldn't drain it for fear of puncturing the expander. After a while it subsided on its own. I felt fine, but that was not going to last long, I knew. Within a few days I was scheduled to start my chemotherapy. It was something I was not looking forward to at all.

8

The Chemotherapy Ordeal

I wasn't convinced six months of chemotherapy was necessary. To me, the operation had ended my problem. It was time to get on with my life. After all, I had already received a healing from God. Why should I put myself through another ordeal?

I prayed for an answer.

Though I received no strong indication from God, I decided to have the chemotherapy. I just didn't feel right refusing it. I felt that if the cancer returned I would regret not doing everything I could to defeat the disease when I had the chance. In fact, if it ever returned I might not be able to do anything about it.

For a long time I had associated chemotherapy with terminal illness. I had never known anyone who had endured the treatment and lived. My experiences with these drugs went back fifteen years to my days as a young nurse working on a medical floor watching cancer patients die a slow, painful death. I'd watch them deteriorate into emaciated, retching, exhausted human beings who succumbed to death after a few series of treatments. I had never worked with individuals who finished their chemotherapy and survived to live to old age free of the disease.

Tremendous advances have been made in the treatment of cancer since I worked on that medical floor. The survival rate is much higher, and the treatment itself less debilitating. But the negative image persisted.

My first treatment came only two weeks after my mastectomy. I was fully recuperated, though, and felt strong as I drove to The Breast Center with Wayne, my mom, and Gladys. I was nervous, naturally, but not overly concerned. Dr. Waisman had assured me the dosage would be small and the side effects minimal.

We chatted about my weekly trip to the center to have the expander filled with saline solution. We talked about the implantation of the prosthesis, which would be in a month or so. We talked easily, not really knowing what we were going to face.

It was impossible, though, for me to keep from thinking about the chemotherapy. I told my family that I was concerned about how I would look and feel during the treatment. Wayne was his usual encouraging self.

"Well, it won't be easy, Beck. But Dr. Waisman doesn't think you'll get very sick. You know the dosage is going to be weak," he said.

"I know. It's just that people look so horrible during chemotherapy." I said, staring out the window at the gray buildings flashing by. "They look like they're going to die."

"It probably seems worse to you because you deal with them at work," he countered. "I don't think I could tell if someone was undergoing chemotherapy."

"You could if they were bald!"

My mom spoke up. "Becky, you know what Dr. Waisman said. There's only about a 10 percent chance you'll lose your hair. Don't worry, honey."

"I know, Mom." I said. "I guess if I can go through childbirth four times I can live through this."

We drove the rest of the way in silence. I was lost in my thoughts until we pulled into The Breast Center's parking lot. We walked slowly across the asphalt and took the elevator to the top floor.

I sat in a daze in a corner of the waiting room staring out the picture window at the people in the parking lot below. I pushed myself back in my seat as if trying to blend into the furniture. I felt like a fearful child left alone at night.

In previous visits to the center, I had seen women sitting in just this manner. At that time I wondered why they were so fearful. Now I knew. I had joined their sad sorority.

When my name was called, I slowly pulled myself from my stupor. I stood awkwardly and walked to the waiting room. Wayne came with me and together we nervously waited for the unknown. I prayed that my fears would be unsubstantiated.

After a few minutes Dr. Waisman entered. He saw how nervous I was and tried to make me feel better. He told me the treatment would probably not be as bad as I thought.

"I want you to relax, Becky," he said, handing me a lemon drop. "It might be unpleasant, but I don't think you'll have any special problems."

"What's this for?" I asked.

"It'll help mask the taste of the chemotherapy."

He then injected an anti-nausea drug into my glutial

muscle before commencing the chemotherapy.

"Please sit over there, Becky," he said, pointing to what looked like a school desk, "and hold out your right arm."

He sat across from me and inserted a hypodermic needle with tubing attached directly into my vein. Then he began to administer the first drug.

The medicine felt hot as it was injected into my arm. Then it felt cold. A sickening metallic taste filled my mouth as if I had bitten into a soft bar of aluminum. My insides were on fire. Then, suddenly, they were freezing. Chills ran up and down my spine. I could feel the drugs course throughout my body.

For the next twenty minutes he injected a number of drugs into my arm through the IV. Some of them were the chemotherapy drugs. Some of them were designed to help alleviate side effects. I could feel each one course through my body. Each one had its own signature.

At the end of the treatment I was helped to my feet. I felt disoriented and nauseous. I was drowsy but managed to walk while someone held me.

After I was led to the waiting room, Wayne took hold of me. I mumbled incoherently as he helped me to the elevator, down to the lobby, across the parking lot, and to the car. He sat me down gently and buckled me up.

I began to nod as we drove. The anti-nausea drug was really taking hold and I had a hard time staying awake. I was even more disoriented than I had been before.

"How many cars are we driving?" I asked, staring with unfocused eyes.

Wayne glanced at me over his shoulder.

"We're only driving one, Beck."

"Oh."

"Are you okay, honey?" my mom asked.

"I'm okay, Mom," I said, in a singsong voice.

It was difficult to focus on the world outside the car window. I sat quietly in a daze. Time did not exist. When we pulled into our driveway, I wondered where we were.

"Are we home already?" I asked.

Wayne nodded.

"Are you sure?"

"I'm sure, Becky."

He opened my door, unbuckled me, and led me into the house. He almost carried me down the hallway to our bedroom. My legs felt like lead and I hung my head down as if it weighed a ton. I mumbled crazy things that no one including myself could understand. My mother told me later that I sounded like a drunken sailor and made about as much sense.

I slept for eight hours, and when I awoke I began retching and vomiting more violently than I ever had in my life. I threw up every half hour for eighteen straight hours with only brief intervals when I could relax and get some sleep. My stomach was cramped and sore, a bitter bile filled my mouth, and the metallic taste continued. I was miserable.

"I can't take this anymore," I moaned to Wayne as I crawled back into bed after throwing up for what felt like the hundredth time. "It's got to get better. I just can't put up with it."

Wayne tucked me into bed and rubbed my cheek with the back of his hand. "Take it easy, Beck. Nobody said it was going to be painless."

"Oh, but not like this. It's not supposed to be like this." I was feeling nervous and jittery all of a sudden, as if I had drunk a dozen cups of coffee.

"Well, maybe the dosage is too strong," Wayne added. "We'll talk to them in a day or so. Just try to take it easy." He looked at me with compassion and worry in his eyes. "I'm sorry it's so rough, Beck, but you've got to tough it out. You've just got to be tough."

I smiled at him and closed my eyes and tried not to think about my sore stomach, which I knew would retch and send me scurrying to the bathroom within a few minutes.

The next day I stopped vomiting. After three days, my head began to clear and I no longer felt queasy. My appetite was gone, though. Every time I ate something I felt the cold bitter taste of metal in my mouth.

Once I started feeling better, my mom and Gladys went back home. They said they'd come back the day of my next treatment and stay for three or four days. They did that again and again until the treatments were completed six months later. On the days they were with us, they ran the household. They cooked the meals, did the laundry, ran errands, took care of the children, and even helped with homework. Because of my mother and Gladys, my children were able to maintain a normal lifestyle throughout my chemotherapy. I don't know what I would have done without them.

Before the second treatment, I had my expander filled with saline solution for the last time. I would have the implant put in within a few weeks. Everything was moving quickly.

I had told Dr. Waisman about my reaction to the first treatment, and he decided to use a different combination of drugs. When I went in for the second treatment, he explained what the changes would be.

"Becky, I think we should try a different anti-nausea

drug," he said, just before giving me the shot. "Part of your problem may be a reaction to the drug. We'll see."

"Anything would be better than before, Dr. Waisman. That was just horrible," I said, shaking my head.

"We'll also give you a tranquilizer with the treatment," he added. "It'll make you relax and help you deal with it a little better. I know it's been rough." He smiled. "Just relax as much as you can."

He injected me with the new anti-nausea drug and then had me sit in the same desk as before. I held out my right arm, and he began the treatment. The doctors never used my left arm because the lymph nodes had been taken from that side and they were afraid that an infection might develop.

I felt the individual drugs surge through my body, first hot and then cold. The metallic taste filled my mouth. I felt tense, and chills wracked my body. It was exactly like the previous treatment.

At the end of the treatment, Dr. Waisman injected the tranquilizer to help relax me during the next few hours. Wayne quickly led me to the car. My head and limbs felt heavy. I was disoriented and talked nonsense.

I didn't talk for very long. Soon after Wayne put me in the car, I fell asleep. The tranquilizer had done its job. My mother told me later that right before I went to sleep, I asked if it were snowing outside. A strange question, considering we were in southern California!

As soon as we got home, I was put to bed. I slept fitfully for a while. When I awoke I began to vomit. I was sick for an even longer period of time than before. I threw up more often and more violently. After an hour or so, I was convinced the cure was more painful than the disease.

A horrible pattern had developed. Following the treatment, I went in and out of a stupor because of the tranquilizers and anti-nausea drugs. Then I was violently sick and disoriented for twenty-four hours. For the next few days I was ill and depressed. Sleeping was difficult. I was hyperactive and confused. After a week, I began to feel better. I was exhausted but not as sick as before. Then I felt fine for a while, but after another week passed, I became anxious and depressed because I knew another treatment was coming up. It was a vicious and almost unbearable cycle. The only positive thing about my ordeal was that I had not gone bald.

During all this, I had the reconstructive surgery done to make me look more natural. It didn't seem possible that I was scheduled to have my third operation in three months, but I was. I didn't dread or fear the surgery, though. In fact, I was looking forward to it.

From the very beginning of my ordeal I had viewed the reconstruction of my breast in a positive light. It was going to make me whole. It was going to make me a normal woman again.

I had confidence in Dr. Handel and the staff at The Breast Center. I was familiar with the procedure and knew what to expect. I was as comfortable as anyone could be when facing surgery.

I was admitted to the day-surgery area of The Breast Center and quickly taken to the operating room. A blood test was taken to check for any changes due to the chemotherapy. After the samples were evaluated, Doctors Handel and Silverstein proceeded with the surgery.

I was anesthetized and the implants were put in place. When I awoke, I saw my new breast for the first time. It was wonderful to be normal again. I felt good about myself and didn't even feel much pain. A few hours after recovery, I was discharged to go home.

The day after the reconstruction, I bought some new clothes. Once again I could wear what I wanted. I could now wear strapless dresses, T-shirts, or even bathing suits. I hadn't realized how self-conscious I had been about my appearance. I felt as if I were reborn.

One month after reconstruction I achieved a major milestone: I went back to work part-time. I wanted to prove to myself that I was normal and that I was capable of being the person I was before I got cancer. I needed to know I could care for my family. I wanted to show myself that I could do my job just as I had before the surgery. For those reasons, it was important to get back to my normal schedule as soon as possible. In a way, I felt that if I could do the things I had done before the surgery I could pretend I never had cancer.

My co-workers responded to me in an almost comical manner. They acted as if I were a china doll—something to be dealt with gently. They spoke quietly and showed me more patience than I wanted or needed. My work load was obviously lightened, and I felt that almost anything I did would be tolerated.

I wanted to be treated like everyone else, but I could see that I would have to make that happen. I didn't want people to be afraid to talk to me about the disease or discuss it behind my back. I decided to be open about the operation in case anyone was curious and wanted to ask.

My physical appearance was also important to me. I had always been well groomed and considered attractive, but now it took on new meaning. I had to show myself and others that the loss of a breast did not make me less of a person or rob me of my sexuality. I became more careful about my makeup and clothing. It was difficult, though, to look good on the outside when on the inside I was suffering from the results of my chemotherapy.

The treatments were still giving me fits. After the third treatment I had taken enough. I had been sick and disoriented for almost twenty-four hours. I was ready to give up.

"I'm through with this, Wayne," I said, while lying in bed the day following my third treatment. "This is ridiculous. I feel like I'm dying. I can't take it anymore. I'm just not sure this is worth it."

"Becky, you need this treatment. You know what can happen if you don't keep with it."

"I can't imagine anything being worse than this. Even cancer couldn't be this bad."

"This is the only protection you have against getting it again," he went on, ignoring my fit of temper.

"I just don't know if I have the strength," I said.

"Look, Beck. You've come a long way. You know how important this is."

"Wayne, it's driving me crazy."

He took a deep breath and exhaled loudly. Then he spoke quietly and calmly, but with conviction.

"You can quit if you want to, Becky. That's your decision. I just want you to know that I think it's a bad idea. I think you should keep taking the treatments to make sure it doesn't come back."

I cried and held him and gave in. But I wasn't convinced. I still questioned the necessity of the chemotherapy.

The rest of that day and the next, I thought about the treatment. I wondered if I really needed to go on. There had been no evidence of cancer in my lymph nodes. Was I putting myself through all this suffering for no reason.

I asked God for help, and once again he heard my plea.

At work the following day, I happened to answer the phone when a co-worker called. She was a friend of mine whose husband had cancer the previous year. Just as in my case, the doctors thought they got it all. It wasn't supposed to spread to his body, so he had no further treatment. She was calling to say the cancer had metastasized, and her husband was now to undergo weeks of intense chemotherapy.

When I hung up the phone, I was convinced God was working in my life again. I knew the call was a message for me. I knew I had to go on for my family, as well as myself.

However, I still couldn't shake my ambivalent feelings about the treatment. I knew I needed it, but I didn't want to face the pain. Did I have the strength to continue.

That's about the time my hair began to fall out.

It was so gradual that at first I didn't notice it. I didn't think much about the few hairs on my pillow each morning or the few strands in my brush. After my third treatment, though, I began to notice the hair in my shower drain and on the bathroom sink. One morning while brushing my hair, I noticed that long strands had fallen out. With each stroke, more and more fell to the floor. I stared at the mirror in horror. My heart sank.

I quickly picked up what little had fallen. As I held the dull and lifeless hair in my hand, I wept. I threw it away in disgust. I tried to deny what was happening to me.

Within a few weeks, the loss was overwhelming. I

refused to brush or blow-dry my hair and washed it only when absolutely necessary. I refused to look in a mirror. Whenever I saw a reflection of myself I felt as if I were staring at a corpse. I was convinced I would end up just like those patients I had taken care of fifteen years before.

All the progress I had made seemed unimportant. It didn't matter that I had overcome the operation. It didn't matter that I was doing something that would help me. It didn't matter that wearing the right kind of clothes could hide my drastic weight loss. My scraggly hair was a constant reminder that I had had cancer.

I soon became obsessed with hair. I thought about it constantly. I compared my stringy thatch to the rich, full hair of others. Everyone around me seemed so healthy and full of life. I felt deathly ill by comparison.

My hair became a tangle of strands, and I could no longer hide the bald spots. I hit bottom and went into acute depression for weeks. I was convinced people knew I had a terminal disease just by looking at me. I dreaded the fact that I might become completely bald. With each passing day I was becoming more withdrawn. I no longer wanted to go outside, and when I did, I wore a hat.

Once again God came to my rescue.

I was sitting in the kitchen one day, lost in my depression, when the phone rang. I got up slowly and answered it unenthusiastically.

"Hello."

"Becky, it's Mom."

"Oh. Hi, Mom."

"Happy birthday."

"My birthday's next week."

"I know, but Gladys and I are coming over today. . . ."

"Mom, I. . . ."

"Now, listen, Beck. We're going to get you a wig for a birthday present," she said. "We think it's a good idea. It'll make you feel better."

I looked out the kitchen window and sighed. I had refused even to look at wigs because that would be an admission that I was going bald. Besides, I had seen wigs on women before, and I thought they usually looked ridiculous. I did not want to go and said so.

"Becky, we're not taking no for an answer. We'll be over in about two hours. Good-bye."

After she hung up, I sat and thought about what she had said. By the time they arrived, I had come around to the idea. However, I still didn't think I could find a wig that would look good on me.

I sat in the back of the car as we drove around the San Fernando Valley looking for wig stores listed in the yellow pages. I was depressed and quiet. Mom and Gladys tried to cheer me up, but it didn't do much good.

We finally found one of the stores we were looking for. I went inside reluctantly, convinced we were making a futile gesture. I was embarrassed because I thought everyone in the store could tell I needed a wig to hide the results of chemotherapy.

I soon changed my point of view.

The first wig I saw caught my eye. I tried it on and was struck by how much it looked like my own hair. Even the style was the same. I felt immediately transformed into my old self. My mother and Gladys and the saleslady raved about the wig and told me how good it looked. We bought it without looking at any of the other models. I hugged Gladys and Mom and thanked them profusely. It was the best present I could have possibly received.

As we drove home, I realized the wig wasn't just a present from Mom and my mother-in-law. I was convinced it was a present from God. It was no coincidence that the first wig I saw was the right one for me. I knew he was still working in my life, and this was one small way of showing me everything would be all right.

Though the wig made me look much better, I was concerned about wearing it in public. I didn't want it to be obvious. That afternoon I practiced wearing it around the house. I combed the hair down across my forehead. I parted the hair a different way. I fussed with it for quite a while.

I wore the wig when I went to pick up the children from school. As we drove home they chatted about school and other children. They hadn't noticed the change.

"How do I look, you guys?" I asked casually, knowing that my own children were my most severe critics.

They sat silently for a moment.

"What do you mean, Mom?" David asked.

"Do you notice anything?"

"I know," Stephen said. "You got your hair fixed."

I smiled, knowing I had passed the test.

"Sort of," I said. "I bought a wig."

We all laughed, and then they told me how good it looked. It was my first real laugh in a number of weeks.

Once again I was comfortable with myself and confident enough to go outside. I no longer thought people could tell I was sick just by looking at me. I felt healthier than I had in a long time.

Of course, I was still a little vain about the wig. Whereas before I wouldn't look in a mirror, I now did. I checked myself in store windows, sunglasses, and anything that provided a reflection. I wanted to make sure it fit properly and hadn't shifted on my head. Strong winds became my enemy.

I was feeling better about myself, but continued to have trouble with the chemotherapy. During the fourth treatment, a new tranquilizer was used. To further alleviate my vomiting, Dr. Waisman prescribed a tranquilizer to be taken every six hours for two days following each treatment. I didn't get quite as sick, but it was still rough.

I continued to have hot and cold flashes as the drugs were being injected. The tranquilizers still knocked me out on the way home. I was still disoriented. The taste of metal was always in my mouth.

Now I was facing a new problem. The tranquilizers that I took at home gave me amnesia. During the time I took them, I had to be watched closely because I would do things and say things that I still don't remember. It was a strange and scary feeling.

I thought that without the vomiting the treatments would be much easier, but they weren't. All the pain and confusion began to add up. I dreaded what I knew I had to face. The week before the fifth treatment I began to get anxious. I cried for no reason and was short-tempered with the family. The day of the treatment was worse. I became nauseous as Wayne drove me to the center. By the time I entered the waiting room, I was a nervous wreck.

Ellen Waisman saw how troubled I was and ushered me into the treatment room. She told me she wanted to talk to me, and that she wanted to help me. I appreciated her concern and was greatly relieved. It was Ellen who finally helped me deal with the chemotherapy.

9

Pac Men, Fire, and Water

"How are you dealing with the treatments, Becky?" Ellen asked as I sat nervously in front of her.

"I'm not getting as sick as I was, but I just don't know if I can take much more."

"Well, that's understandable," she said. "I know it's very unpleasant, but it is getting better."

"I don't think you really do know, Ellen," I answered, feeling tired and scared about what I was going to face. "You may deal with these patients all the time, but you've never gone through it. It's horrible, and I can hardly bear it." As bad as I felt, I tried not to take it out on Ellen. She had been good to me. The entire facility had been good. I tried to be strong, but I was feeling miserable.

"I know I've never experienced it, Becky. But I think I can help. I feel for what you're going through."

I stared at her blankly.

"I think you should see a counselor, Becky. She may help you deal with your anger and your fear a little better. They're really making progress with visualization and relaxation techniques."

"I don't want to see a counselor. I don't need one. Besides, I don't think I have the time. It's difficult enough to arrange my trips for the chemotherapy, let alone counseling." I told her I could deal with it in my own way.

"You know, Becky, I think you should see the chemotherapy as a friend, not an adversary."

"A friend?" I asked incredulously. "How can I see it as a friend? It makes me sick as a dog. It wrecks my body, makes me crazy. How can I see that as a friend?"

"It's helping to save your life."

"Are you sure?"

"Why else go through with this?"

"I don't know."

I really didn't know. I didn't know what to tell Ellen. I didn't know how she could help. I knew I was being difficult and stubborn but I could do little about it. I was not showing my faith in God very well. I was not really dealing with anything very well.

"I appreciate all the help and guidance that's available," I said, "but I've been too busy trying to survive the whole thing to really study anything new or see it a different way."

"I can understand that, Becky. But you know, this is the turning point. After this treatment you're more than halfway through."

Her words seemed to turn a switch in my mind.

"I guess that's right, isn't it? I hadn't even thought about that."

"Well, I think it's a good way to look at it. The worst part is behind you."

When I received my chemotherapy that day I realized I was one step closer to my goal. However, it was still agonizing. I cried throughout the treatment and felt victimized by the drugs.

After the effects of the treatment wore off, I considered what Ellen had said about seeing the chemotherapy as my friend. Maybe visualization and relaxation techniques could help me deal with my problem. I remembered a time while I was still in nursing school when a counselor used those very same techniques to help some of my patients. The patients sometimes fell asleep during the sessions; even I felt drowsy a couple of times. Perhaps I could use the techniques to help me through the last half of the treatments.

I started reading books about patients who had survived cancer, and I noticed a pattern to all the success stories. Everyone who survived the disease had used visualization and relaxation techniques. I read some books on these techniques, but I still wasn't sure how they could help me.

I attended a class that Ellen recommended at The Breast Center. It mainly covered tips on skin care and how to hide the effects of the chemotherapy. It was also an unofficial support group.

During the class, we'd share our experiences and talk about how we were dealing with our problems. It was healthy to open myself to other women who had suffered as I had. I always left feeling good.

A number of women in the class were using visualization and relaxation techniques. They talked about how they actually pictured the death of the cancer cells. The class instructor told us that it was this visualization that really helped her deal with chemotherapy. Their experiences reinforced what I had read. I decided at last to use the techniques myself.

I still had misgivings about visualization, though, and before I began, Wayne and I talked it over.

"I think it might be very effective," he said one evening after the children were put to bed.

"I know, honey. But it seems like I wouldn't be putting my trust in God."

He looked at me. "I guess I never thought of that."

"Do you think it's stepping beyond the bounds of faith?"

"God gave you your mind, Beck. I'm sure he'd want you to use it."

"That's true."

"I don't think there's anything wrong with it. If it'll help, I'm sure God would want you to do it."

"It can be like a prayer," I said. "Like a meditation on God."

Wayne nodded and smiled. "I think that'd make it even more effective."

"But, you know, they're giving me all these drugs to keep the cancer away. It seems silly to try to just think it out of my body."

"Well, everybody seems to agree that it helps. The doctors, the women at the class, they think it helps. You should do all that you can. I think God would want you to use anything available to make sure that cancer doesn't return."

"I think you're right, Wayne. Everything I've read indicates that it helps. It sure helped the women in my class."

He nodded.

"I think I'll start."

"The hard part will be finding a quiet place in this madhouse to do it," he said jokingly.

I laughed, knowing full well how right he was.

The next day I got a relaxation tape to help me with my visualization. That night, after putting the children to bed and making sure they were asleep, I asked Wayne to listen to the tape with me.

We took off our shoes and sat on opposite sides of the couch. The soft voice on the tape told us to close our eyes. Then it said that we'd be tightening and loosening a series of muscle groups, beginning with our face and working on down the body. We were told to tighten and loosen the muscles in our forehead. Then the voice told us to do the same with the eyebrows and the muscles around the eyes.

I was just starting to relax when I heard Wayne snoring from across the room. I tried to focus on the tape but couldn't. I started laughing and soon realized I wouldn't be getting anything from the tape that night.

"Come on, Wayne," I teased as I awakened him. "We might as well go up to bed. I'm going to have to do this by myself from now on, I guess."

Though it came naturally to my husband, the relaxation wasn't easy for me. I had a hard time getting into the proper state of mind for the visualization. Of course, having four children running around the house wasn't much of a help. It was weeks before I could concentrate enough not to be disturbed by someone entering the room or making noise nearby. Once I reached that state of mind, though, the technique worked well.

As the weeks progressed, I slipped into a pattern. Three times a day—morning, noon, and night—I'd listen to the eight-minute tape and then begin my visualization. It was becoming part of my battle armor in the war with cancer.

"What do you think about when you do it, Beck?" Wayne asked me one evening after I finished my exercise.

"Well, I sort of copied what others did. Some people saw their white blood cells as soldiers killing the cancer. Some viewed the chemotherapy like a vacuum cleaner, sucking the cancer cells into a disposable bag. Others visualized Pac Man gobbling up the cells."

"Pac Man?" he teased. "I was expecting something a little more original."

I shrugged. "It works."

"So what do you do?"

"I start with my relaxation, and then I do my deep breathing. I think about how God breathed life into Adam. I picture Jesus breathing life into me."

"That's great," he said, smiling.

"Then I picture him giving me a big breath which purifies the blood that's rushing through the walls of my lungs."

"You actually see these things."

"I picture it as well as I can, yes." I answered. "After that, the purified air goes through my lungs to my heart and then to my other organs, cleaning them all. I do that all through the body, three or four times."

"And the kids don't bother you? You don't get disturbed?"

"Not much anymore. I've really improved."

"It's like Genesis," he said. "Where God formed man from dust and breathed into his nostrils the breath of life."

"Yea," I agreed. "I guess I'm also receiving the breath of life."

I told him that I then visualized billions of tiny white cells marching through my body with scrub brushes and magic cancer-killing spray, cleansing every bone and organ."

"It's hard to believe you can see all that."

"Well, it's taken a great deal of practice and concentration, but, yes, I do see it. I had to change the visualization frequently until I finally found what worked well for me."

"I'm so glad it does, Beck." He hugged me and told me he was proud of what I had accomplished.

Over time, I changed a few things. Sometimes I'd picture my white blood cells like Pac Men. Instead of gobbling up cancer cells, they used a spray bottle and rag to spread an anti-cancer juice, making sure the disease didn't return. I made sure the little Pac Men cleaned everything the blood could not quite purify. When they were finished, I had the Pac Men put the rags into a double red bag like the ones that are used at hospitals to dispose of toxic materials and throw them out of my body, along with normal bodily waste.

I decided to try visualization to help me cope with the chemotherapy itself. I convinced myself the drugs were a positive force in my life, not something negative. In the days before my next treatment, I visualized the heat of the drugs as a fire burning the cancer from my body. I viewed the cold chills as a mountain stream washing away all the dead cells.

I practiced the relaxation and visualization the morning of my sixth treatment, and to my amazement there were no tears or fear. It was difficult to maintain control, but I closed my eyes and concentrated. The session was over before I realized it.

I was even better prepared for the seventh treatment. My relaxation and visualization had become a daily ritual. I also decided to start an exercise program. As soon as the amnesia lifted following my seventh treatment, I rode my bicycle daily. It helped clear my head and made me feel physically stronger.

During my eighth treatment, Dr. Waisman commented on how much better I was dealing with the chemotherapy.

"You sure have a better attitude toward it now, Becky," he said as he was preparing to give me my eighth dosage.

"I can hardly believe what I was like before. You must have thought I was crazy carrying on like that."

"No, we didn't think you were crazy. We know how tough it is. You didn't act any different from anybody else, really." He paused for a moment. "But there's no more tears now."

"No, the visualization and relaxation are really helping. I feel like part of the team," I joked.

"The most important part," he said.

Of course, all of my problems weren't over. I was still having trouble with the chemotherapy. It was still unpleasant.

One of the most disagreeable side effects was the horrible taste that the chemotherapy left in my mouth. It affected the taste of my food. Everything I ate tasted like the drugs. Even chocolate, which I loved, was tainted by the chemotherapy.

I tried a number of things to take the taste of chemo out of my mouth. I sucked on mints and hard candy. I also chewed gum.

However, I had to be selective with the gum and candy. One evening at work I chewed some gum to get the foul taste of a recent treatment out of my mouth. The taste of the drugs instantly filled my mouth. I threw out the gum and sat down for a moment, trying to relax. I couldn't understand why I was suddenly feeling so sick. The feeling passed as soon as it came on, and only later did I realize that it was the gum that made me ill. It had the same flavor I had chewed just after the injection of the drugs. I associated the taste with being ill, and chewing the same gum again brought back the nausea. From that point on I continuously changed brands to avoid that problem.

Due to the tranquilizers, I continued to have amnesia following each treatment. It felt strange to have my loved ones tell me some of the things I did and said. I couldn't remember a thing.

My mother told me that following one of my last treatments, I staggered downstairs, made some tea, and sat down to the morning paper. I had done that countless times in the past, but this time I was reading it upside down.

A short time later I announced that I was going to ride my bike until I burned the drugs out of my body. Gladys managed to dissuade me, but I insisted on at least taking a walk. I put on a hat, walked across the street, tripped on the curb, returned to the house, and fell asleep on the couch.

The following day I couldn't remember what I had done. My family wisely decided to keep me in the house whenever I began to act irrationally. It was a sound idea.

I certainly did some strange things. Some of them even seem funny now, but at the time they scared me deeply. I did not like doing things I wasn't aware of. Sometimes I felt I was losing my mind.

I worked hard at getting well. I continued my visualization and relaxation. I continued to ride my bike and read God's Word daily. Now, though, I added the last piece of armor in my defense against cancer.

In my reading I discovered the correlation between diet and breast cancer. A diet of fatty foods could make one more vulnerable to the disease. Because of that, I decided to change the family's eating habits.

I found that with a little creativity, I could make interesting meals that were high in fiber and low in fat. This was important for Wayne and me, but it was especially important for the children. Cancer tends to run in families. Therefore, my children were statistically more likely to get the disease than those whose parents never got cancer.

The day I had been anticipating for six months finally arrived. I was to receive the last dose of drugs. As we drove to The Breast Center, I felt eager and excited to conclude the treatments.

When I arrived, I stepped into what seemed like a celebration. Everyone who was involved in my care greeted me and congratulated me. Dr. Waisman and his staff nurse, Sherry, hugged me and told me how pleased they were that I had finally reached the end of my ordeal.

I was led to the treatment room for the last time. I sat in the desk. As Sherry prepared the IV, I stared into her eyes.

"I will never need this again," I said emphatically.

She smiled and agreed. Then I closed my eyes and began my visualization as Dr. Waisman began injecting the drugs. As I felt them surge through my veins, I visualized fire burning the cancer from my body, then a cold mountain stream washing away the dead cells.

10

On to Recovery

A number of factors contributed to my successful encounter with cancer. My faith in God, strong family ties, a healthy attitude, fine medical care, and other factors enabled me to survive the disease. Each of them played an important role.

Faith in God was the backbone to my sanity. I knew that only God could give me the strength to go on. Christian friends from Canada to Mexico prayed for my recovery. I could feel their strength and support. Christian brothers and sisters were constantly preparing meals, sending cards, offering to care for my children, or helping in any way possible. God worked in my life in a powerful way.

The support of my mother, my mother-in-law, my sisters, my husband, my children, and the rest of my family and friends made all the difference in the world. They're the ones who held my hand after I discovered I had cancer. They drove me to the center and sat with me during my diagnosis. They did my chores after my surgery. They provided strength for me during the treatments. They were always there.

My mother and mother-in-law were especially important. They worked together every three weeks for six months to make sure our household continued in a relatively normal manner. Things would not have been the same without them. Their contribution cannot be overstated.

The medical care I received was also a major factor in my recovery. The Breast Center is a fine institution with the latest technology to help women overcome breast cancer. Their skilled physicians and counselors made survival possible. I trusted them completely, and I will always be indebted to them for their care and understanding.

Of course, my own attitude helped. Once I got over the shock and horror of knowing that something was growing inside me, I decided to take an active part in my recovery. As soon as I quit feeling sorry for myself, the real work could begin. I read about cancer, particularly breast cancer, to find out all I could about the disease. I slowly began to develop a positive attitude toward recovery. I read the Bible daily. I continued my visualization and my low-fat, high-fiber diet. I also continued to exercise daily. These things worked together to make me stronger spiritually, mentally, and physically.

All who follow these guidelines will help themselves in the battle against cancer. Not all battles can be won, but they all can be fought courageously. Life can be extended for days, weeks, months, years, and can be made more meaningful. That may be just as important.

Of course, there was a lingering fear that the cancer may return. After my chemotherapy was over, I still wasn't convinced that I had whipped it completely. The month between my last treatment and my first post-cancer checkup was a difficult time. Every ache and pain scared me: I was afraid the cancer had returned. I was almost nostalgic for the days when I had my monthly treatment. At least then I could count on regular meetings with my doctor and assurances that all was well.

Those four weeks seemed like an eternity. When I finally went back to the center, I was assured that my fears were normal and that I was healthy. That was quite a relief.

I have slowly learned to listen to my body. If it's tired, I rest it. If it is tense, I ride my bike or get away and relax. I push all negative thoughts from my mind, and I eat a well-balanced diet. I thank God that after twenty-four months I remain free of cancer, and I feel and look wonderful. I'm in good shape, I eat better, and my hair has grown back even fuller than before.

I know God has helped me, and I pray that my life may be an inspiration to others who try to carry their burdens alone. Christ said in Matthew 11:28-29, "Come to me, all you who are weary and burdened; and I will give you rest. Take my yoke upon you and learn from me, for I am gentle and humble in heart, and you will find rest for your souls." I believe those words with all my heart because, without the help of God, I would have never survived my bout with cancer.

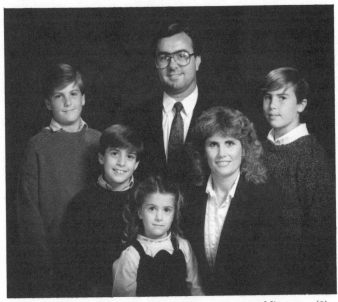

Becky's family in 1988. From left: Stephen (11 years old), Aaron (8), Aimee (5), Becky's husband (Wayne), Becky, and David (13).

The Authors

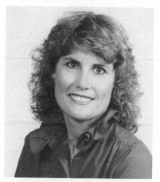

Becky Lynn Wecksler

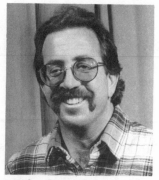

Michael Wecksler

Becky Lynn Wecksler was born in Riverside, California, in 1951. She married her high school sweetheart, Wayne, in 1971 and graduated from nursing school in 1972. She and her family reside in Saugus, California.

Becky continues her nursing career working part-time in the recovery room for a rural trauma center, Henry Mayo Hospital, Valencia.

Most of her days are spent juggling time between the activities of her school-age children: David, Stephen, Aaron, and Aimee.

Becky became a Christian shortly before the birth of her first child. She presently teaches Sunday school for the first through third grade at Faith Community Church in New-hall and is also in charge of their helps ministry.

Michael Wecksler was born into an American family in Wiesbaden, Germany. After high school in Riverside, California, he spent seven years working odd-jobs and traveling extensively in Canada, the United States, and Mexico. Before finishing college, he lived in Colorado, Hawaii, Oregon, and Washington.

Wecksler worked for two years as the editor of a small weekly newspaper in northern California, then struck out on his own as a free-lance writer. Though he focuses mainly on fiction, he has had articles published in *Discovery* and *New Words* magazines.

Wecksler lives with his wife on five forested acres near Mt. Shasta. He has recently finished his first novel and is working on his second, as well as a collection of short stories.

Michael is Becky's brother-in-law. *In God's Hand* is Becky's story as told to Michael.